PRAISE FOR *THE O.*

Dr. Scheele, who has proven credentials as an eminent scientist, has the gift of revealing the intricacies of normal and defective functioning of the body. In this book he presents, in a manner understandable to non-scientists as well as experts, his discovery of the biological basis of weight control and metabolic health.

Dale Bockman, MD
Professor of Pathology
Medical College of Georgia

This well-written and readable book delivers - in its early chapters - a critical assessment of the history and the current state of obesity research. In later chapters, Dr. Scheele draws on his own research findings to make a compelling case for a new paradigm for weight control. Readers will come up with new ways of looking at, and fighting, unhealthy weight gain.

Dario B. Valenzuela, PhD, MBA
Biotechnology Professional

Drawing upon decades of emerging research, The Obesity Cure *begins with historical accounts of weight loss regimens, continues to cross-cultural comparisons of diet, to considerations of modern dieting plans, and finally culminates in a new concept called "Selective Protein Deficiency Syndrome." As such* The Obesity Cure *is a revolution in the understanding of the interplay of sugars, proteins, and fats, and how they contribute to weight control. Dr. Scheele's book has the precision of a rigorous scientific work but one which is delivered in a way that is accessible to everyone.*

Lilly Zhang, M.D.
Lenox Hill Hospital/LIJ, New York, NY

Dr. Scheele came to the world of nutrition after years of experience focused on digestive enzymes in some of the most renowned institutions in the United States. In his recent book, The Obesity Cure, *Dr. Scheele proposes that deficiencies in the food chain lead to an imbalance in metabolic pathways that affect regulation of body weight. Based on extensive laboratory and human studies, he formulated a novel therapeutic regime of power amino acids (essential, positively-charged and satiety amino acids) that tame appetite and correct for deficiencies in the food chain to improve metabolic health and normalize body weight. The thoughtful and original contributions presented in* The Obesity Cure *are not only impressive but most welcome in this highly visible and important area of weight control and human health.*

Alan M. Tartakoff, PhD
Professor of Pathology and Director of the Cell Biology Program
Case Western Reserve University
Cleveland, OH

In this groundbreaking work, Dr. Scheele presents new metabolic concepts that shed valuable light on the current epidemic of obesity and poor metabolic health in America. In a facile manner he shows us how to restore metabolic health and normal body weight with the power of essential and positive charged amino acids – "power amino acids."

Paul Webster, III, M.D.
Former Chairman, Department of Medicine
Medical College of Georgia
Augusta, GA

As a Professor who has published with several Nobel laureates, I found Dr. Scheele's new book, The Obesity Cure, *a breakthrough in understanding metabolic disease and obesity. Every single page provides critical information to fully explain how dietary foods can "make" or "break" body health.* The Obesity Cure *explains how a deficiency in positive-charged amino acids, proteins and metabolic pathways can lead to metabolic disease and further how Power Amino Acids can correct for these deficiencies improving overall body health by harnessing the body's natural feedback mechanisms to regulate appetite, metabolic rates, and body weight.*

George Pieczenik, PhD
Professor of Molecular Biology
Rutgers University

As a registered nurse who has a strong interest in nutrition for the prevention and treatment of disease, The Obesity Cure *has opened a brand new path toward healing. The way that Dr. Scheele discusses obesity and other metabolic diseases that are associated with the Metabolic Syndrome is unique and unequaled in this cluttered field. The way the author has connected deficiencies in the food chain with diet-related metabolic diseases, including obesity, is masterful. Nutritional science has not fully appreciated the role of essential, positive-charged and satiety amino acids in human health. As such many people will benefit from the discoveries revealed in this book and will live to see improved health in their own private lives.*

Joanne Paller, RN
Aiken, South Carolina

There are very few books that have the potential to change one's life like The Obesity Cure *authored by Dr. Scheele, one of the eminent scientists in today's world. Dr. Scheele is masterful in explaining the essentials of dietary health and the importance of supplementing the diet with power amino acids that correct for the deficiencies in amino acids, proteins and metabolic pathways that occur due to deficiencies in the food chain. Thanks to Dr. Scheele, this new field of essential amino acid nutrients has been opened wide for all to see. Does it work? You betcha! Everything he predicted in his book has happened to me for the better, even after retiring. I feel better than I have ever felt in the past 40 years. If you do yourself one favor this year, buy* The Obesity Cure *and reclaim your health with Power Amino Acids!*

Stanley Naskiewicz
Howell, New Jersey

Chapters 4 through 7 discuss how the body changes energy pathways through hormonal mechanisms as food substrates (carbohydrate, fat, and protein) change in the diet. We learn that hormones regulate fuel utilization (fat-burning versus carbohydrate-burning) in a manner that is largely all-or-nothing. When the body is burning carbohydrates, it shuts down the metabolism of fats. We learn that carbohydrate metabolism takes precedence over fat metabolism. These discussions allow us to understand that a food industry that enriches numerous products with refined sugars and produces foods that are brimming with excessive carbohydrates and fat promotes overweight disorders.

Chapter 8 teaches us that overweight disorders are only one dimension of a wide spectrum of metabolic diseases that are caused by nutritional excesses. We learn that the harmful effects of excess dietary carbohydrates include free radical formation, oxidative stress, protein glycation, advanced glycation end-products, and inflammatory processes that not only lead to overweight disorders but also to cardiovascular diseases, cancer, and other chronic diseases that are associated with the Metabolic Syndrome, accelerated aging and early death. In Chapter 9, we pause to reflect on the numerous paradoxes that abound in the world of nutritional health, even after we understand the deleterious effects of excess dietary carbohydrate.

The second half of the book reveals a missing part of the equation that may explain the "weight loss paradox," that quizzical dilemma that occurs during aging when overweight individuals cut back on food intake but cannot lose weight, whether they exercise or not. "Selective protein deficiency syndrome" is introduced in Chapter 10 as the missing concept in understanding the caloric equation that controls body weight. We learn, for example, that protein health is required to repair the body and rebalance the metabolic pathways that burn fat and restore core body health. We learn that selective protein deficiency syndrome in the presence of excess carbohydrate diets leads to excessive weight gain in experimental animals. This chapter teaches us that there is a vulnerability in the food chain for 9 essential amino acids, which are required for continuous protein synthesis but are not produced by mammals, including human beings. We further learn that a dietary deficiency of essential amino acids, which we call "power amino acids," leads to deficiencies in positive-charged proteins and metabolic pathways that lead to unwanted weight gain and poor metabolic

Book Overview

In Chapter 1, "The Great Divide in American Diets," we learn that neither low fat/protein, high carbohydrate diets nor high fat/protein, low carbohydrate diets, as tested over the past 100 years, is sufficient to achieve that elusive goal of sustained weight control and metabolic health, especially in our current culture of food abundance. Something appears to be missing in our understanding of weight control. There seems to be a missing piece of the puzzle that, if discovered, might resolve, once and for all, the challenge of avoiding both the unwanted weight gain that becomes progressively more problematic during the aging process and the chronic degenerative diseases that lead to untold suffering.

This book is dedicated to revealing the "missing piece" that might allow us to direct our weight-loss efforts toward more effective control of body weight and metabolic health. That "missing piece" appears to be the presence of "selective protein deficiency syndrome," a newly identified condition that seems to limit the capacity of the body to alter the metabolic pathways that control weight gain and loss. Based on 35 years of emerging scientific and medical discovery, "selective protein deficiency syndrome" appears to provide the new concept, the "secret" if you will, that may allow us to achieve the elusive goal of sustained weight control.

In order to reveal the full story and place all the pieces of the puzzle into correct alignment with one another, this book is structured along the following lines. The first half of the book focuses on the enormous progress that has been made over the past 50 years in understanding the metabolism of carbohydrates, fat, and protein. During this time, much has been learned about carbohydrates and their harmful effects on body health when consumed in excess. To understand these harmful effects, we discuss, in Chapter 2, the concept of "diseases of civilization," which was introduced by epidemiologists who studied isolated populations around the globe in the early part of the 20th century. In Chapter 3 we discuss how the body has learned, through evolution, to adapt to changes in the environment, including the ever-changing availability of foods on a daily basis, by modulating the expression of enzymes (proteins) that drive metabolic pathways.

- *High fat/protein, low carbohydrate diet:* the forward slash indicates that the diet contains high fat and high protein
- *Low fat/carb, high protein diet:* the forward slash indicates that the diet contains low fat and low carbohydrate
- *Carb:* this designation is occasionally used in this book for carbohydrate
- *Selective Protein Deficiency Syndrome:* this syndrome (SPDS) is presented as a new entity that describes the continuum that exists in protein deficiency disorders between normal function and Kwashiorkor, which represents a far-advanced form of protein deficiency that presages early death in underdeveloped countries. SPDS is discussed in detail in Chapters 10 through 14 and distinguished from Kwashiorkor in the Notes section for Chapter 10

"It is not the critic who counts. The credit belongs to the man who is actually in the arena; whose face is marred by the dust and sweat and blood; who, at the best, knows in the end the triumph of high achievement, and who, at worst, if he fails, at least fails while daring greatly; so that his place shall never be with those cold and timid souls who know neither victory or defeat."

– Teddy Roosevelt

- How we feed personnel in the military
- How we feed individuals who are suffering from chronic degenerative diseases associated with poor metabolic health
- How we feed aging seniors
- How we feed the elderly in nursing homes

They will change the fundamental nutritional concepts in America and change the food profiles in grocery stores, health food stores, drug stores, and convenience stores. They should fundamentally change the way Americans eat in today's sedentary culture. And, they may revolutionize the treatment of eating disorders (such as anorexia nervosa, bulimia and chronic fatigue syndrome) in the advanced world.

Finally, these new concepts should also revolutionize the treatment of malnutrition in the under-developed world.

An End As Well As a Beginning

Just as the Roman God Janus reminds us that any gate or door may be traversed in two directions, the revolutionary new concepts revealed in this book may be seen both as an end to the paradox of weight control and as a beginning in understanding how such weight loss concepts may be implemented and further studied. On the one hand, implementation of these new concepts needs to be promoted in the medical and nutritional communities. On the other hand, nutritional and biochemical scientists need to further determine the role of essential amino acids and positive-charged proteins in body metabolism, including not only the control of appetite and the metabolic pathways that regulate fat storing and fat burning pathways but also the anti-aging factors that lead to increased longevity with improved quality of life.

Definition of Terms

The terms that will be used in this book to describe individual diets and new concepts are as follows:

- *Low fat/protein, high carbohydrate diet:* the forward slash indicates that the diet contains low fat and low protein less increases protein deficiency, which causes catabolic reactions, loss of muscle tissue, and further loss in the capacity to burn fatty acids.

This book will resolve the weight loss paradox, and other paradoxes as well, in ways that are simple to understand and easy to implement. The solution to the weight loss paradox is amazingly simple: supplementation with power amino acids.

Search for the Answer

Knowing the solution to the Weight Loss Paradox set me on another mission. Surely, someone must have formulated the correct treatment for protein deficiency and excess weight disorders. I checked in the grocery stores, the health food stores, the drug stores, and the convenience stores. What a letdown it was when I discovered that components of the remedy could be found in several individual products, but the optimal formulation was nowhere to be seen!

It is then that I formulated the optimal remedy for relieving or combating protein deficiency associated with overweight conditions, obesity, Type II Diabetes, and Metabolic Syndrome. Naturally, this remedy contains power amino acids. It also contains other essential nutrients including vitamins, minerals, micronutrients and protein.

My original quest to improve America's health provided critical information not only on weight loss and weight control but also critical information on other health concerns. Consequently, the final chapters of this book focus on metabolic health, revitalized youth, and aging health and reveal how people supplemented with power amino acids achieve anti-aging health that may lead, not only to increased comfort, satisfaction, and well-being, but also to increased longevity with improved quality of life.

The Dream

The novel concepts about weight control presented in this book are so fundamental to nutritional health they will revolutionize the prevention and treatment of obesity in America. They should also revolutionize:

- How we feed our children during growth and maturation
- How we feed individuals in the prime of life

More than likely, they may benefit by taking dietary supplements to meet their needs for essential amino acids.

◊ Nonessential amino acids are of lower value. Since the body synthesizes these amino acids, we are less concerned that they be present in the diet or food chain.

◊ The public has a good understanding of essential fatty acids. However, it has very little understanding of the importance of essential amino acids.

Because protein deficiency plays an important role in overweight conditions and obesity, there is a need to understand the importance of essential amino acids in:

- Unwanted weight gain
- Cellular starvation and catabolic states
- Production of positive-charged proteins that lead to nutritional and body health
- Correction of protein deficiency states that lead to obesity
- Resetting of body metabolism from fat storage to fat burning pathways
- Stimulation of weight loss and lasting weight control
- Maintenance of health and the prevention of diseases during the aging process.

Because of the critical importance of essential amino acids and positive-charged proteins in weight control, health, nutrition, and aging, we now refer to essential amino acids as "Power Amino Acids" and to optimal health, with the full complement of positive-charged proteins and negative-charged proteins, as "Supercharged Health." For example, supplementing the diet with "power amino acids" confers "power nutrition" and "supercharged health" on overweight individuals and primes the body for weight loss and lasting weight control.

The Weight Loss Paradox

There is a significant paradox in current weight loss strategies and regimens. The usual prescription is to eat less to lose weight. However, eating

- Protein deficiency leads to catabolic states that break down muscle tissue. With less muscle tissue, people have less capacity to burn fat.
- Protein deficiency in cells reduces the synthesis of positive-charged proteins first, which dramatically impairs metabolic pathways and nutritional health. In essence, many of the working units (enzymes) in cells throughout the body disappear. To use a sports team metaphor, one is no longer playing with a full team of proteins or enzymes. Because of the role that enzymes play in body metabolism, metabolic pathways are no longer balanced throughout the body. And without balanced metabolic pathways, body health is severely compromised. As health declines, the prospects for disease and aging dramatically increase.

This book explains, in simple language, how protein deficiency impairs or blocks weight loss and weight control. Specifically, the book explains the following new concepts:

- The difference between protein substrates (protein calories) and fuel substrates (sugar, carbohydrate, and fat calories):

  ◊ Protein substrates in the diet are considered high-value foods because, in addition to providing energy, they restore nutritional health to the body. On a cellular level, nutritional health includes production of all of the proteins (working units) that confer optimal health and nutrition.
  ◊ Fuel substrates in the diet (sugar, carbohydrates, and fat) are considered low-value foods because they are used chiefly as sources of fuel for energy demands. As such, they are critical for energy and locomotion. However, if more fuel calories are ingested than burned, these calories act as "empty" calories. As unburned, empty calories, they may rapidly lead to obesity.

- The difference between essential and nonessential amino acids:

  ◊ Essential amino acids are of higher value. Since the body does not synthesize them, they must be acquired from the food chain. This means people must eat foods enriched in essential amino acids.

of obesity and its treatment. However, at the time, it was not clear that the results in experimental animals could be extended to humans.

Focus on the Obesity Epidemic in America

By now it was the Third Millennium, and I had entered the world of entrepreneurs. In 2000, I founded NovaLife, which develops health-care and nutritional products. Throughout the 1980s and 1990s, an epidemic of obesity had emerged with increasing impact in the United States. By 2004, 64% of Americans were declared overweight, and 32% qualified as obese. Furthermore, many of my friends seemed to be afflicted by the Metabolic Syndrome, which, although poorly understood, describes a common syndrome in aging individuals, characterized by weight gain, hypertension, increasing cholesterol levels, and numerous chronic degenerative diseases associated with aging.

Could I now combine all of the information that I had discovered on protein, carbohydrate, and fat metabolism, relate it to nutritional health, and figure out how to treat overweight conditions, obesity, and the Metabolic Syndrome? Could I now focus on the obesity epidemic to improve health in America? Could I possibly go further and improve health around the globe?

The medical world understands that obesity results from excessive carbohydrate and fat intake in a sedentary society. However, nutritional scientists and medical doctors do not agree on simple, effective strategies for stimulating weight loss and achieving lasting weight control.

A Startling Discovery: The Role of Protein Deficiency in Obesity

Based on extensive personal research on obesity demographics tracked from 1900 to 2000, I have found, in addition to increased food intake and decreased exercise, the following new relationships:

- From 1900 through 2000 our diets have become progressively enriched in refined sugars.
- From an analysis of the nutritional traps that lead to overweight conditions and obesity, the common thread is protein deficiency.
- People who eat less food to lose weight become more deficient in protein.

first time, the molecular signals that direct proteins to secretory compartments in the cell. This work was recognized in the 1999 Nobel Prize in Medicine awarded to Dr. Blobel, my second mentor.

With hard work, these inventions allowed me to make quantum leaps in scientific discovery and to help define the cutting edge in cell biology and protein chemistry. But what about my mission to improve health in America?

Focus on Nutrition and Health

These same inventions allowed my laboratory at the Rockefeller University and colleagues at the Philipps University in Marburg, Germany, to study nutritional health as a function of protein, carbohydrate, and fat levels in the diet. Our studies determined how changes in the diet resulted in changes in digestive enzymes secreted from the pancreas. For example, higher protein in the diet stimulated the pancreas to make increased amounts of enzymes that digest proteins in the intestinal tract. Similar investigations studied variations in carbohydrate and fat in the diet. Taken together, these studies, conducted over two decades, showed how Pavlov's dietary adaptation in the pancreas is regulated by specific intestinal hormones.

When our focus was switched to the study of protein deficiency in the diet, we made a number of startling observations that led to scientific breakthroughs in understanding the deleterious effects of protein deficiency on weight control, nutritional health, and ultimately aging health as well.

As we restricted protein in the diet, we initially expected that the quantity of all proteins in the body (the pancreas in this respect) would slowly diminish. However, we found a completely different response. Positive-charged proteins decreased by 90%. In contrast, negative-charged proteins showed no decrease. This imbalance in protein synthesis apparently allows the body to survive for longer periods of time but greatly impairs the health of the organism.

In the presence of protein deficiency and increased carbohydrate levels, the weight of experimental animals increased by 30% in 12 days! Although it had not been our initial intent, we inadvertently had discovered an animal model of dietary obesity that correlated with both carbohydrate excess and protein deficiency. With impairments in protein health, the body apparently resets its metabolic pathways to store fat. Furthermore, by increasing the protein in the diet and decreasing the carbohydrate, we observed loss of weight in these animals. Thus, in the laboratory, we had solved the paradox

Proteins as the "Working Units" of Life

Along this academic route, I developed a strong interest in proteins and began to appreciate that proteins are the "working units" of the body. Unique as enzymes, proteins are the only molecules that actually do work in the biological world. They are like construction workers at a building site: they frame the building, apply the wall boards, and drive the nails. Within the body, proteins are unique in other ways as well. They are three-dimensional folded structures with distinct shapes. With complementary surfaces, proteins fit together in multi-protein complexes and assemblies. In the presence of membranes, they give rise to intracellular organelles and whole cells. In higher life, cells join together to form multicellular organisms, including human beings.

As enzymes, proteins show specific activities; with activities, proteins have behavior; with behavior, proteins show personalities. On a molecular level, one can recognize the identities of individual proteins as easily as one recognizes Aunt Mary or Uncle John in real life!

Inventions and Scientific Discoveries

At each turn in the road, I invented new scientific procedures, which allowed innovative scientific discoveries at the cutting edge of science and medicine. My development of "Pancreatic Lobules" as a robust model of cellular secretion allowed my laboratory to define how digestive enzymes were secreted from pancreatic cells in response to hormones and neurotransmitters.

My invention of the two-dimensional gel electrophoresis procedure allowed my laboratory to be the first to separate human, mammalian and rodent proteins in high resolution and, therefore, chart the movement of the complete set of digestive enzymes through intracellular compartments in glandular cells. 2D gel electrophoresis ushered in the era of "proteomics," the high-resolution study of proteins and protein function, twenty years before that term was coined by the scientific community

Together, with the work of others, my discoveries were recognized in the 1974 Nobel Prize for Medicine that was awarded to Dr. George E. Palade, my first scientific mentor.

Work with intracellular organelles (dog pancreatic microsomal membranes in particular) allowed Günter Blobel and me to define, for the

Introduction

The story of this book actually began far from the Pyramids of Giza and the tombs in the Valley of the Kings. The story began in the West shortly after I graduated from Johns Hopkins Medical School, during my years of training as an intern and resident in internal medicine. Although I was highly trained as a medical doctor and cared deeply about my patients, my dedication turned quickly into a dream and a question. My dream was to improve the health of America. The question was "where could I start to accomplish my dreams"?

Instead of treating individual patients for their personal medical problems, why not find the cures for individual medical diseases so that all patients throughout the country and possibly the world could benefit? Without knowing the particulars of my quest, I knew it would take hard work, further education, and an intense desire to make new medical discoveries. I wanted to work on a major unmet medical need. In short, I wanted to fix something big and help the world in doing so!

My quest for doing something important was not new. My visual talents allowed me to think big! I could see everything in three-dimensional space, even in my imagination. I could see detailed landscapes of cities I had previously visited around the world. I could visualize landscapes of organs and tissues throughout the body. In time I would be able to visualize how individual proteins formed complexes within cells, how proteins improved health, and how nutritional health promoted weight loss and control.

These visual talents gave me an edge that allowed me to advance, with time, from Washington-Lee High School in Arlington, VA, first to Princeton University, then to Johns Hopkins Medical School, The Osler Medical Service at Johns Hopkins Hospital, The University of California at San Francisco, The Rockefeller University, Yale University School of Medicine, and Harvard Medical School, the last three as Professor.

Although I was truly thankful for his advice and greatly benefited from his service, I would not fully understand the nutritional lesson for another thirty-five years. At the time, I could not fully comprehend how a Bedouin in the desert sands of Egypt could teach me a lesson that I had not learned from my western education!

However, with the wisdom and humility that comes with age, it now seems that not only might I benefit, but many other of my fellow Americans might benefit as well from new lessons on nutrition that may allow us to treat America for the nutritional diseases, including over-weight disorders and obesity, that have reached epidemic proportions in this country.

My First Lesson in Nutrition

It is surprising how I received my first lesson in nutrition. As a native born American who received an Ivy League education and was fortunate to attend one of America's top Medical Schools, you might think that my lessons in nutrition would come from the hallowed halls of Johns Hopkins Medical School, which I attended in the early 1960s. Or, you might think that such a lesson would have been learned during internship or residency training on the Osler Medical Service at Johns Hopkins Hospital or possibly during my last year of residency training at the University of California, San Francisco Medical Center, in the late 1960s.

Yet there I was in Egypt on a trip to visit the Pyramids of Giza, those impressive tombs built for Egyptian leaders who lived and ruled millennia ago. I traveled by boat up the Nile River to Luxor, a resort town located close to the Valley of the Kings. Intent on visiting the tombs of King Tut (Tutankamen) and others, I hired a guide to take me to these ancient treasures. I was disappointed when the guide showed up with a donkey because my heart was set on riding a camel into ancient history. After a few minutes of discussion and negotiation, my guide disappeared into the streets of Luxor and returned with a camel. I was delighted, and so we set forth to explore the tombs in the Valley of the Kings.

Within a couple of hours, riding in the hot Egyptian sun without sunscreens that would be developed later, I was thoroughly dehydrated and exhausted. We visited a primitive desert Inn for lunch before visiting these historic treasures. Outrageously thirsty, I asked the owner for an iced-cold cola. I drank it straight down and asked for another. It seemed I could drink six colas. At this point the owner, who was very knowledgeable on such things, advised me that colas, with their high sugar content, do not quench thirst, in the hot desert climates of Egypt, or anywhere else for that matter. (Later I would learn that each 12 oz cola contains 30 grams of sugar.) Instead, he recommended that I drink lemon juice squeezed into a glass of water. I followed his instructions and was amazed to find that my thirst was immediately quenched!

Contents

For Peoples Around The World

Whatever Your Calling

May You Have The Gift of Understanding:

The Highest Priority in Life is Good Health

HUMMINGBIRD

The hummingbird, with bright plumage and exotic colorations,
is an ancient symbol of health in the western hemisphere.

THE OBESITY CURE: Weight Control, Metabolic Health, Revitalized Youth with Power Amino Acids

ePDF ISBN   978-0-9825708-0-7
ePUB ISBN   978-0-9825708-1-4
Print ISBN   978-0-9825708-2-1

For information, contact:

   NovaLife®
   7825 Fay Avenue, Ste. 200
   La Jolla, California 92037
   www.factor4health.com

Power Amino Acids® and FACTOR4 Weight Control® are registered trade marks of George A. Scheele, M.D.

THE OBESITY CURE

Weight Control, Metabolic

Health, Revitalized Youth with

Power Amino Acids

George A. Scheele, M.D.

NovaLife®
San Diego, California

health. We validate this new concept by showing that 96% of overweight human subjects lose weight when treated with a supplemental regimen of power amino acids.

In Chapter 11 we formulate a general theory of nutrition and weight loss health that links power amino acid supplementation to metabolic health, weight control, revitalized youth, and anti-aging health. This theory explains how the early phases of protein deficiency, and more specifically selective protein deficiency syndrome, together with the harmful effects of excess carbohydrate, may lead, to metabolic disturbances that result in the Metabolic Syndrome, which is associated with a number of chronic degenerative diseases, including overweight disorders and obesity, type 2 diabetes, cardiovascular disease, certain forms of cancer, and other diseases that were originally classified as diseases of civilization. We define a new concept, called "supercharged health," which occurs when power amino acid supplementation corrects nutritional deficiencies in amino acids, proteins, metabolic pathways, body health, and aging.

Chapter 12 provides the arguments that power amino acid supplementation is superior to high-protein foods and protein supplements in improving the four cornerstones of human health—weight control, metabolic health, revitalized youth, and anti-aging health—that lead to increased longevity and improved quality of life. Chapter 13 provides practical advice on using power amino acid supplementation together with restrictions on intake of refined sugars, complex carbohydrates, and saturated/hydrogenated fats to lose weight and regain the metabolic health that promotes the four cornerstones of human health and happiness. Chapter 14 discusses the world potential for supercharged health and argues that by achieving the four cornerstones of human health around the globe, worldwide productivity may be increased on an exponential scale.

By identifying the missing piece in our understanding of the dietary principles required to achieve sustained weight control, this book allows us to take a revolutionary step beyond the high fat/protein diets of pioneers like Dr. Robert Atkins and the low fat/protein diets of public health policy. For perhaps the first time, we can define a low fat/carb diet that produces significant weight loss without the starvation protocols that lead to catabolic (destructive) health and extreme hunger. The missing piece revealed in this book is the importance of the dietary supplementation of essential and positive-charged amino acids ("power amino acids") that maintain anabolic (constructive) health and at the same time achieve feelings of comfort, satisfaction, and well being that are associated with natural appetite suppression. This book further explains in detail why power amino acids are superior to high protein foods and protein supplements for achieving the weight-loss health that restores the body to a more youthful physique and the improved metabolic health that combats the chronic degenerative diseases that often result in accelerated aging and early death. On a practical level, the book shows how this new information may be easily incorporated into the dietary habits of individuals all across America to optimize energy storage and use to minimize obesity as well as many of the other diseases that are associated with the Metabolic Syndrome.

Part 1

Dietary Studies over
the Past 100 Years

"Truth, like beauty, when unadorned, is adorned the most."

– William Beaumont

Chapter 1

The Great Divide in American Diets

The story could not have been better. He was one of the best-trained doctors in America. He was highly motivated to relieve suffering and disease. More than anything, he wanted to stem the rising tide of heart disease in America. He was on a mission, and no one could stop him. His medical pursuits in the late 1940s and early 1950s had provided the answer. In the mid 1950s, he suggested that eating fat and cholesterol caused heart disease and probably obesity as well. His efforts to prevent disease changed public policy in the United States for years to come.

His name was Ancel Keys. Like other achievement-oriented men, his life was shaped by the events of his time. The allies were winning World War II, first on the European front and later on the Pacific. The involvement of the United States made the difference and turned the tide in this global conflict. As Tom Brokaw writes in *The Greatest Generation*, America was spawning great heroes. There was almost no challenge that Americans could not take on and win! This included the challenge Ancel Keys took for his own, the challenge of revolutionizing American health.

Following World War II, Dr. Keys turned his efforts to the war against cardiovascular disease and overweight disorders.

The National Consensus on Dietary Fat and Cholesterol

By 1950, it was already well known that cholesterol was one of the primary components of the atherosclerotic plaques that cause cardiovascular disease. In the late 1940s, laboratory rabbits given a diet high in cholesterol developed atherosclerotic plaques throughout their arteries. Within a few years, the same phenomenon was observed in chickens and dogs. It seemed natural to assume that heart disease in humans might begin with the abnormal accumulation of cholesterol-containing plaque in arterial walls and that the accumulation of plaque might be caused by excessive levels of cholesterol in the blood circulation. Linking serum cholesterol with heart disease and obesity became the focus of Key's life.

In the early 1950s, medical technology was still relatively primitive, and only rudimentary techniques existed for studying heart disease in humans. What Keys and his colleagues needed was a way to measure cholesterol levels. When Rudolph Schoenheimer and his colleagues at Columbia University developed the first assay for measuring cholesterol levels in the blood stream[1], Keys was off and running.

With his wife, Margaret, a medical technician, Keys correlated dietary customs with the incidence of cardiovascular disease on a global scale. As Ancel and his wife traveled around the world, Margaret would measure total cholesterol in the blood and Ancel would survey total fat in the diet. Keys compared cholesterol levels and mortality rates from heart disease in the United States, Canada, Australia, England and Wales, Italy, and Japan. From these comparisons, Keys formulated his hypothesis that diets rich in fat and cholesterol gave rise to cardiovascular disease and obesity.

Keys concluded that the ideal diet for healthy hearts would increase the percentage of carbohydrate calories from less than 50% of calories to almost 70% and reduce the proportion of fat calories from 40% to 15%.[2]

Table 1-1

	Carbohydrate	Fat	Protein
Normal diet	<50%	40%	>10%
"Ideal" diet	70%	15%	15%

Key's ideas on cholesterol and heart disease were novel and persuasive. In 1958, *JAMA* (the *Journal of the American Medical Association*) wrote that, "the most reasonable diet to employ for weight reduction is one that maintains normal proportions of fat, protein, and carbohydrate and simply limits the total quantity of the mixture." The American Heart Association (AHA) embraced Key's cholesterol theory in December 1960, when it accepted a short report stating that "reducing the fat in their diets and replacing saturated fats with polyunsaturated fats" would reduce the risk of heart disease. Shortly thereafter, *Time Magazine* put Keys on its cover as the face of dietary wisdom and authority in America. The low-fat/low-cholesterol diet was becoming part of an unquestioned orthodoxy.

The Big Picture

In his recent book, *Good Calories, Bad Calories,* Gary Taubes traced the efforts of Keys and other investigators over the past 100 years to develop diets that would control weight and disease in the advanced world. His book is without equal in its thorough examination of conflicting opinions among authorities. His research included interviews with over 600 clinicians, investigators, and administrators. The riveting and compelling story challenges the conventional wisdom on diet, weight control, and disease. Much of the historical material in the next few chapters is based on his masterful book that sets the stage for understanding why the medical establishment has misunderstood the impact protein health has on nutritional health and weight control in modern society. These impacts will be the subject of later chapters in this book.

Low Fat/Protein Diets (Semi-Starvation Diets)

Ancel Keys first became interested in dietary studies and health during World War II. Epidemiological studies conducted during World Wars I and II showed that food shortages of a few years' duration coincided with dramatic decreases in the incidence of heart disease to about one-fourth of previous rates.

In 1944, Keys and his colleagues at the University of Minnesota studied the physiological and psychological effects of starvation associated with war. Over nearly six months, 32 conscientious objectors consumed semi-starvation diets of 1,570 calories per day and followed that with up to 20 weeks of rehabilitation. The high-carbohydrate, low-protein, and low-fat diet consisted mainly of whole white bread, potatoes, cereal, turnips, and cabbage, and only minimal amounts of meat and dairy, while the number of calories allowed was approximately half the calories that the subjects had been accustomed to. Keys calculated that subjects on this diet should lose an average of 20% of their body weight.

While the subjects did lose weight during the first 24 weeks, the results were catastrophic in other respects. Every subject complained constantly about a continuous gnawing sensation in the stomach, a clear symptom of hunger. The men experienced decreases in blood pressure and pulse rate. They suffered from anemia, an inability to concentrate, and marked weakness during physical activity. They complained of weakness, loss of ambition, narrowing of interests, depression, irritability, loss of libido almost to the point of obliteration, and feelings of growing old.

The men slowed down, cutting the amount of energy they expended by more than half. Five subjects developed character neuroses and two individuals developed psychoses. When the subjects were allowed to resume eating normally during the rehabilitation period, they remained prodigiously hungry. They consumed up to 8,000 calories a day without losing their hunger. At the end of rehabilitation, subjects carried, on average, 5% more weight and 50% more body fat than they had carried before the study began.

National Health and Nutrition Examination Surveys

Starting in the 1960s, the federal government began periodic surveys of Americans to study their health and nutrition, and particularly to monitor obesity and the other risk factors associated with heart disease. Since then, four National Health and Nutrition Examination Surveys (NHANES) have documented an alarming rise in national obesity. Until the early 1970s, up to 14% of Americans were obese. By the 1980s, this figure had risen to 20%; by the early 1990s, it was approximately 30%. While obesity rose in all segments of the population, it was particularly a problem for those low in income and education. The usual explanation is obesity became a social problem during the 1970s, when Americans, for the first time, began consuming more calories than they burned.

Public Policy Recommendations

As we will see, the dietary-fat hypothesis of Ancel Keys was based on incomplete information. Nevertheless, it was widely embraced by both doctors and the public. In the early 1970s, the U.S. Department of Agriculture (USDA) issued dietary guidelines to keep Americans healthy and fit. Not surprisingly, its recommendations were predicated on Keys' theories. In 1976, Congressional hearings directed by South Dakota Senator George McGovern also concluded that dietary fat was responsible for cardiovascular disease and obesity. And in 1982, the National Academy of Science report, *Diet, Nutrition and Cancer,* reinforced the proposition that dietary fat caused cancer and cardiovascular disease by recommending that Americans cut fat consumption even more drastically than previous recommendations, to levels of 30% or less.

In 1986, *JAMA* published the results of a Multiple Risk Factor Intervention Trial (MRFIT) study conducted by Jeremiah Stamler. In this study, Stamler plotted death rates against serum cholesterol levels and concluded that the association between cholesterol and heart disease applied to *any* level of serum cholesterol[3]. Thus, according to this study, everyone would benefit from lowering serum cholesterol levels. In 1987, the National Cholesterol Education Program (NCEP), established by the National Institutes of Health (NIH), recommended that total cholesterol should be below 200, a conclusion that was echoed by the National Institutes of Health Consensus Conference, organized by the National Heart, Lung and Blood Institute (NHLBI).

It may well be true that high serum cholesterol levels contribute to cardiovascular disease. However it does not follow that lowering dietary fat is the only way to lower serum cholesterol levels. Nevertheless, Surgeon General C. Everett Koop's 1988 *Report on Nutrition and Health* admonished Americans to reduce dietary fat. A year later, the National Academy of Science threw its weight behind the same conclusion. In *Diet and Health: Implications for Reducing Chronic Disease Risk,* it stressed that reducing fat intake be given the highest priority. No more than 30% of calories should come from fat and no more than 10% of calories should come from saturated fat.

In 1991, under the guidance of Dr. Bernadine Healy, the first female Director of the National Institutes of Health, the NIH began a $700 million project, the Women's Health Initiative, to study the connections between dietary fat and both cancer and cardiovascular disease. Forty-nine thousand women between the ages of 50 and 79 were enrolled in the study, which lasted nearly a decade. Twenty thousand were put on a low-fat diet and compared to a control group of 29,000, who continued to eat their normal diets. Women on low fat diets were encouraged to eat more vegetables and fruit, as well as fiber in the form of whole grains. The intent was to limit dietary fat to 20% of their calories. On average, these women lowered their daily intake by 360 calories.

The final results were disappointing. At the end of almost 8 years, participants weighed, on average, only two pounds less than they weighed when they started. Their waist circumference, a gauge of abdominal fat, actually increased. Investigators who supervised the WHI reported in 2006 that subjects who ate the presumed "healthy diet" low in fat, high in fiber, and high in vegetables, fruits, and whole grains had no less heart disease, stroke, breast cancer, or colon cancer.

The steady barrage of public policy statements from various governmental agencies spawned an entire generation of diet doctors who prescribed low-fat/protein, high carbohydrate diets. The "Dean Ornish Diet" was one of the most strict, prescribing diets with 10% fat. Government agencies and the medical establishment were intent on winning the war against cardiovascular disease and obesity, and they added cancer as well to the list of diseases they thought they could prevent with a low-fat diet.

Key's hypothesis was supported by numerous authoritative government agencies and committees: the McGovern Committee, the Surgeon General, the National Academy of Science, the USDA, the MRFIT study, and the National Institutes of Health Consensus Conference and its National Cholesterol Education Program. Collectively, they consistently disregarded annoying evidence to the contrary. Only the data that confirmed the consensus hypothesis were emphasized.

As we will see, cholesterol levels represent only the "tip of the iceberg." In medical terms, cholesterol levels form what may be called an "epiphenomenon": although it is a component of lipoprotein particles and involved in lipid transfer throughout the body, cholesterol is neither the central nor the main cause of fat deposition and atherosclerosis. Cholesterol, however, was the first lipid component to be subjected to diagnostic examination. The early association between total cholesterol levels in the serum and cardiovascular disease and death gave rise to an incomplete and incorrect understanding of the causes of atherosclerotic disease and obesity.

It would take another 50 years for medical science to work out the basic details of the mechanisms involved in the development of cardiovascular disease. And much still remains to be discovered before we can have a complete understanding of the mechanisms, including those that give rise to overweight disorders and obesity.

Shift from Cholesterol to Fat and Heart Disease to Obesity

During the late 1980s, the focus brought to America's health shifted. It began when increasing numbers of questions were raised about the narrow concentration on cholesterol. Several nagging discoveries raised questions about Keys' conclusions:

- Critics noted that Keys based his conclusions on an analysis of data from only six countries, even though data were available for 22 countries. When all 22 countries were included in the analysis, the apparent link between cholesterol and heart disease vanished.
- Keys found no measurable differences in the cholesterol levels of male subjects who were fed diets high and low in cholesterol for a period of months.
- David Rittenberg and Rudolph Schoenheimer demonstrated that dietary cholesterol accounts for only 20% of cholesterol in our blood. The liver produces the rest.
- A 24-year heart study conducted in Framingham, Massachusetts by Thomas Dawber and associates found no relationship between cholesterol and sudden cardiac death.
- While the MRFIT data showed a modest increase in male death rates when serum cholesterol increased from 157 to 250 and a sharp increase when serum cholesterol increased from 250 through 281, a reanalysis of the MRFIT data in the 1990s also showed an *inverse* relationship between cholesterol and both stroke and premature death. Men with very low cholesterol levels were also prone to premature death. Below 160 mg/dl, the lower the cholesterol, the shorter the life.
- During the 1990s, Japanese investigators reported that fat intake in Japan had increased from 6% in the 1950s to 22% as the Japanese diet changed to include progressively more milk, meat, fish, and shellfish. While cholesterol levels increased from 150 to nearly 190 mg/dl (compared to the average American cholesterol level of 202 mg/dl), the changes were accompanied by a remarkable reduction in the incidence of stroke, a reduction in the incidence of deaths due to heart disease, and no change at all in the prevalence of heart disease.

- Between the late 1970s and the late 1990s, the World Health Organization had studied heart disease and risk factors around the world. Its MONICA study (MONItoring CArdiovascular disease) had examined the heart attacks and medical records of almost 6 million men and women in numerous populations living in 21 countries. It concluded that mortality from heart disease everywhere was declining, and neither cholesterol levels, blood pressure, nor smoking habits could explain the decline.
- The "French Paradox" associated with the Mediterranean diet suggests that nations consuming high-fat diets show remarkably little heart disease.
- In 1990, the National Heart, Lung and Blood Institute organized a workshop to discuss the relationship of low cholesterol and high mortality. Men whose cholesterol levels exceeded 240 were at greater risk of premature death because of increased risk of heart disease. In contrast, men with cholesterol levels below 160 were more likely to die prematurely from cancer, respiratory and digestive diseases, and trauma. However, the cholesterol associations with heart disease appear to be distinctly different between men and women. For women, it appeared that the higher the cholesterol the greater their longevity.

Further, it became clear that calorie consumption in America was on the rise. Between 1971 and 2000, in spite of longstanding public policies to encourage weight loss by restricting fat in the diet, the average weight of Americans had steadily increased. American men had increased their calorie consumption by an average of 150 calories per day. Over the same period of time, women increased their consumption by more than 350 calories per day. The Centers for Disease Control (CDC) attributed this caloric increase "primarily...to an increase in carbohydrate intake." It is significant that the CDC did not attribute this weight gain to fat consumption. Fat intake did increase by 50 calories in women. But, average fat intake in men actually decreased by 50 calories over this same period of time.

The USDA reported in *Nutrient Content of the U.S. Food Supply, 1909–1997* that the number of calories the average Americans consumed each day rose from 3,300 in 1971 to 3,800 by 1997. Given that a normal diet traditionally consisted of 2,500–3,000 calories a day, these statistics show that the increase in calorie consumption was dramatic in a relatively short period of time. However, the percentage of fat in the diet *fell* over this same period of time, while protein intake remained the same, marginally low. Of the additional calories available for consumption each day, fully 90% came from carbohydrates.

Data from the Centers of Disease Control in 2002–2004 show that 22.7% of adults nationally were obese. Even more disturbing, the percentage of people who are overweight and obese continues to increase year after year. Since 2004, the figures for obesity and overweight disorders have climbed to 32% and 64%, representing nearly one-third and two-thirds of Americans, respectively. The status of overweight disorders and obesity is measured by the body mass index (BMI), which is defined as body weight in kilograms divided by height in meters squared. Adults with a body mass index of 30 or more are considered obese. Those with a BMI between 25 and 30 are considered overweight. This equation works for almost everyone except weight lifters.[4]

Shelley Hearne, Executive Director of the Trust for America's Health says, "bulging waistlines are growing, and it's going to cost taxpayers more dollars regardless of where you live. We have a crisis of poor nutrition and physical inactivity in the U.S. and it is time we dealt with it." Health policy analysts point out that obesity increases the burden on taxpayers, because public policy requires Medicare and Medicaid programs to cover the treatment of disease caused by obesity. Taxpayers spent $39 billion in 2003 for the treatment of conditions associated with obesity.[5]

Yet the picture gets worse. The *Annals of Internal Medicine* reported in 2005 on an investigation of 4,000 people studied over three decades. Over the study period, 9 out of 10 men and 7 out of 10 women become overweight. Not even those who made it to middle age without getting fat were safe. Half of the men and women in the study who had made it into adulthood without a weight problem ultimately became overweight. One third of the women and one fourth of men became obese.

As the long-running Framingham, Massachusetts study has shown, obesity raises the risks of heart disease, cancer, diabetes, arthritis, hypertension, and elevated cholesterol levels. These results more than demonstrate that overweight conditions and obesity are diseases of increasing desperation that lead to multiple chronic degenerative diseases and early death.

Human Studies on Obesity

In the 1970s and 80s, Jules Hirsch used semi-starvation diets on obese subjects monitored on metabolic wards at the Rockefeller University. Eventually more than 50 subjects who lived at the Rockefeller University Hospital underwent intense metabolic studies related to fat intake, distribution, and storage. For 4 weeks of baseline metabolic studies, patients ate a normal diet. They were then shifted to a 600-calorie liquid formula and studied during the ensuing months for loss of weight. As patients lost weight, the overriding question was whether fat cells shrank or disappeared. A secondary question was whether patients who lost weight could maintain their weight loss after returning to a "normal diet." By utilizing state-of-the-art metabolic studies, Hirsch assumed that the mechanisms of weight gain and loss could finally be understood.

Although it could not be fully determined whether fat cells disappeared or shrank in size, adipose tissues (fat storage sites) did significantly decrease during the semi-starvation diets. However, once they returned to a normal diet, all of the patients regained the weight they had lost, and some regained more than they had lost.

The greatest surprise of all was that metabolic activity, measured according to energy expenditure per square meter of body surface, dramatically changed as a function of calories absorbed into the body. When their calories were restricted, subjects reduced their energy expenditure and metabolic activity disproportionately. When they consumed more calories, their metabolic activity increased, again disproportionately. Studied after their weight loss, subjects burned up to 24% fewer calories than individuals who were naturally thin.

Ethan Sims, at the University of Vermont, studied the reverse during the 1970s. What would happen if thin people who never had a weight problem got fat? A group of male prisoners was used for this study. Once the men got fat their metabolism increased by 50%. They needed more than 2,700 calories per square meter of body surface to stay fat but needed just 1,800 calories to maintain their normal weight. When the study ended, the prisoners had no difficulty in losing weight. Within months, they were back to their normal weight and effortlessly stayed there.

Albert Stunkard, of the University of Pennsylvania, knew from population studies that obesity appeared to have a genetic component. Eighty percent of the offspring of two obese parents become obese. No more than 14% of the offspring of two parents of normal weight become obese. He used the Danish Registry of Adoptees to study whether body weight is inherited. In this registry, adoptions occurred very young. For example, 55% of adoptees had been adopted in the first month of life, and 90% were adopted in the first year.

Stunkard's conclusions from these studies were that:

- adoptees were as fat as their biological parents, and
- how fat they were had no relation to how fat their adoptive parents were

A second study used data from the Swedish Registry of Twins. In this registry 93 pairs of identical twins were reared apart; 154 pairs of identical twins were reared together; 218 pairs of fraternal twins were reared apart; and 208 pairs of fraternal twins were reared together. The study concluded that identical twins had nearly identical body weights and body mass indexes (BMI), whether they had been reared apart or together. At the same time, fraternal twins showed large variations in body weight and BMI.

Taken together, these results suggest that genetic influences are important in body fatness and further suggest that childhood family environment alone has little or no effect. Body weight is more strongly inherited than nearly any other condition, including mental illness, breast cancer, or heart disease.

Each person appears to have a comfortable weight range within which the body gravitates. The range might span 10 or 20 pounds. However, going much above or below the weight range seems to be difficult. The body resists drastic weight change by increasing or decreasing the appetite and by changing the metabolic rate to reset the weight back to "normal."

As important as these studies are, they do not take into account the distribution of calories among carbohydrate, fat, and protein. As we will see, however, those are crucial distinctions. Understanding the importance of the composition of the diet, whether it is a high carbohydrate, low protein diet or a high protein, low carbohydrate diet, is critical to understanding the dynamics of weight loss.

Low Fat/Protein, Semi-Starvation Diets Do Not Work

By the third millennium, after 50 years of misaligned public policy, it has become abundantly clear that low fat/protein, high carbohydrate diets under conditions of caloric restriction do not result in weight loss.

The Cochrane Collaboration is a volunteer network dedicated to studying the effects of healthcare interventions. In 2002, it reviewed semi-starvation diets and concluded that low-fat diets were no more effective in producing weight loss than low-calorie diets, both of which produced results that were "so small as to be *clinically insignificant.*"

In 2001, the U.S. Department of Agriculture had come to the same conclusion after its review of 28 relevant trials of low-fat diets. Twenty of these were also calorie-restricted diets that allowed up to 1,700 calories a day. Over a 6-month period, subjects averaged not quite nine pounds of weight loss. The subjects of the one year-long study reduced their caloric intake to 1,300 calories for 18 months. They emerged from the study, on average, one pound heavier than when the study began!

George Thorpe, a Kansas doctor who chaired the AMA's Section on General Practice and treated obese patients himself, claimed that semi-starvation diets would inevitably fail, because they worked "not by selective reduction of adipose deposits, but by wasting of all body tissues, including muscle."

Laboratory Animals Grow Fat on High Carbohydrate Chow

In 2001, Paul Zimmet reported in *Nature* that the Israeli sand rat, when removed from its native habitat and given an abundant, high carbohydrate diet, "…develops all of the components of the Metabolic Syndrome, including diabetes and obesity." Sprague Dawley and Wistar rats will also routinely become overweight after 6 to 12 months on similar laboratory chow in a caged environment. Purina chow for rodents, for example, contains 49.4% carbohydrates, 23.4% protein, and 3.8% fat; it is abundantly high in carbohydrate and low in fat.

Caged monkeys will also become obese and diabetic on similar diets. In a 1965 study by John Brobeck of Yale, Rhesus monkeys became fat and mildly diabetic on Purina Monkey chow, which contains 59% carbohydrate.

In this case, not only was the diet high in carbohydrate, but it was also marginally low in protein.

Persistence of Public Policy

Despite overwhelming evidence that semi-starvation diets fail to achieve the intended weight loss, current medical orthodoxy continues to recommend semi-starvation diets for losing weight. According to the 1998 *Handbook of Obesity*, edited by George Bray, Claude Bouchard, and W.P.T. James, "dietary therapy remains the cornerstone of treatment and the reduction of energy intake continues to be the basis of successful weight reduction programs."

In *Good Calories, Bad Calories*, Gary Taubes summarized his conclusions about the 60-year medical romance with semi-starvation diets. "Over the course of a century, a paradox has emerged. Obesity, it has been said, is caused, with rare exceptions, by an inability to eat in moderation combined with a sedentary lifestyle. Those of us who gain excessive weight consume more calories than we expend, creating a positive caloric balance or a positive energy balance, and the difference accumulates as excessive pounds of flesh. But if this reconciles with the equally 'indisputable' notion that 'eating fewer calories while increasing physical activity are the keys to controlling body weight,' as the 2005 *USDA Dietary Guidelines for Americans* suggest, then the problems of obesity and the obesity epidemic should be easy to solve." However, as Taubes points out, low fat/protein, high carbohydrate diets prevent neither cardiovascular disease nor obesity.

High Fat/Protein Diets

Now that we have examined the paradoxical results with low fat/protein diets, we need to examine the results of high fat/protein, low carbohydrate diets. Fortunately, there is no dearth of data to examine, as Taubes points out.

The story of high fat/protein diets starts out with Blake Donaldson in the 1920s and 1930s. Donaldson had spent a full year trying and failing to reduce weight in obese patients. Then, he learned from anthropologists at the American Museum of Natural History in New York City that prehistoric humans lived almost exclusively on "the fattest meat they could kill." Based on this evolutionary argument, Donaldson selected seventeen thousand patients and treated them over four decades with a high fat diet. Because fat tends to follow protein and exclude carbohydrate, these diets were likely high in fat and protein and low in carbohydrate. Most of Donaldson's patients lost 2 to 3 pounds per week. And those who did not lose weight appeared to have a "bread addiction."

Although Donaldson never published his observations, he shared his results with his colleagues at New York Hospital. Apparently, in the audience that day was Dr. Alfred Pennington, who was sufficiently convinced to try the diet himself in 1944 and to prescribe it for his patients as well.

While working for E.I. du Pont de Nemours and Company after World War II, Pennington tested a high fat/protein, low carbohydrate, unrestricted caloric diet on overweight DuPont executives. The 20 executives fed this meat-rich diet lost between 9 and 54 pounds and averaged nearly 2 pounds per week. Not only did the executives not experience hunger between meals, but they reported "increased physical activity and sense of well being."

Pennington's diet consisted of 3,000 calories and restricted carbohydrates to no more than 80 calories per meal. Pennington reported that even this much carbohydrate prevented weight loss. One Du Pont executive lost 62 pounds on the diet and kept it off for more than two years, all the while consuming 3,300 calories of meat a day. However, if he ate "even an apple," Pennington wrote, his weight would increase. In 1954, Pennington reported his studies in the *American Journal of Digestive Diseases*: "Here is a treatment that, in its encouragement to eat plentifully, to the full satisfaction of the appetite, seemed to oppose not only the prevailing theory of obesity but, in addition, principles basic to the biological sciences and other sciences as well."[6,7]

In 1985, George Blackburn and Bruce Bistrian administered a diet in which 50% of the calories came from protein and 50% from fat to 700 patients. The average patient lost 47 pounds over a period of 4 months. This translates to an equivalent of almost 3 pounds per week.

In 1980, John La Rosa reported that measurable weight loss without hunger occurred in a number of high-protein, high-fat diets that ranged from a low of 1,000 calories, through a mid-region of 1,400 or 1,800 calories, a normal range of 2,200 calories, and a high count of more than 2,700 calories. The same results occurred repeatedly, even when patients were "encouraged to eat as much as necessary to avoid feeling hungry" but to avoid carbohydrates while they did that.

Role of Carbohydrate in High-Protein, High-Fat Diets

Based on observations between 1963 and 1973, Robert Kemp made three observations: his obese patients craved carbohydrates; they did not understand why other people could remain thin on the same diet; and they were puzzled why they had once eaten the same diet themselves, at an earlier age, and remained thin. Kemp formulated a "working hypothesis that the degree of tolerance for carbohydrate varies from patient to patient and indeed in the same patient at different periods of life." Then he developed a carbohydrate-restricted, calorie-unrestricted diet that he said made it "possible for the first time to produce worthwhile results in obesity treatment."

As recently as 2003, physicians from Yale and Stanford Medical Schools published a consensus report "on the efficacy and safety of carbohydrate-restricted diets." They examined 38 such diets. Of these, 34 produced greater weight loss than diets higher in carbohydrates. On average, restricting carbohydrates to 60 grams a day produced 37 pounds of weight loss, compared to a weight loss of 4 pounds when carbohydrates were not restricted.

The Atkins Diet

Alfred Pennington's high fat/protein, low carbohydrate, eat-as-much-as-you-like diets are now more commonly recognized as the Atkins diet, based on Robert Atkins, the author of *Dr. Atkins Diet Revolution*. Robert Atkins was trained as a cardiologist at Cornell Medical Center in New York City. As a young physician in the early 1960s, he gained 50 pounds. Atkins had read Edgar Gordon's article in *JAMA*, "A New Concept in the Treatment of Obesity." In this article, Gordon had claimed that a diet high in protein and fat but limited in carbohydrates to measured amounts of fruits, green vegetables, and minimal bread would produce weight loss without complaints of hunger.

Atkins modified the Gordon diet by increasing Gordon's initial 2-day fast to a week or more of strict carbohydrate limitation. After first losing a reported 28 pounds in a month and feeling an increase in his own energy, Atkins administered his diet to 65 junior executives at A.T.&T, all of whom had noticed his dramatic weight loss. All of them showed similarly dramatic decreases in weight loss.

Atkins' Diet Revolution

Atkins then began to treat overweight subjects and wrote his initial book on the *Diet Revolution*. He began the program with an initiation period during which patients were to eat no carbohydrates except for two small, green salads a day. After the introductory phase, patients were instructed to add carbohydrates gradually back into their diet until their weight loss leveled off or reversed. They were instructed then to cut back on the carbohydrates until their weight loss resumed. Because weight loss forced the body into a state of ketosis, Atkins instructed his patients to use ketosticks to measure the ketone bodies in the urine that signaled weight loss was occurring.

Once women's magazines began promoting his diet in 1966, Atkins' business boomed. In 1970, *Vogue* popularized his diet when it published an article entitled, "The Famous Vogue Superdiet Explained in Full."

Atkins' Dream

Atkins wanted to start a revolution, not just create a diet. "Just as Martin Luther had a dream," wrote Atkins, "I too have one. I dream of a world where no one has to diet. A world where the fattening refined carbohydrates have been excluded from the diet." Atkins claimed that his patients lost "thirty, forty, 100 pounds" eating "lobster with butter sauce, steak with Béarnaise sauce…bacon cheeseburgers…" Atkins further wrote, "As long as you don't take in carbohydrates, you can eat any amount of this 'fattening' food and it won't put a single ounce of fat on you."

Atkins' Summons

Eventually Atkins encountered the wrath of the medical world. The American Medical Association sponsored a denunciation of the Atkins diet in 1973 in an article written by Theodore Van Itallie. Jean Mayer wrote in his syndicated newspaper column that "The American Medical Association has taken the unusual step of warning the U.S. public against the latest do-it-yourself diet as propounded in 'Dr. Atkins Diet Revolution.'"

In the same year, Atkins was summoned to appear before George McGovern's Senate Committee on Nutrition and Human Needs. Three medical experts were summoned to testify against Dr. Atkins. They charged that the Atkins diet was neither revolutionary, nor effective, nor safe. Fred Stare of the Nutrition Department at Harvard (who did not appear in person), sent the following statement, "The Atkins diet is nonsense. Any book that recommends unlimited amounts of meat, butter and eggs, as this does, in my opinion is dangerous. The author who makes the suggestion is guilty of malpractice."

Dr. Atkins countered at the hearings. "It is incredible that in twentieth-century America a conscientious physician should have his hard-won professional reputation placed on the line for daring to suggest that an obesity victim might achieve some relief by cutting out sugars and starches."

Ketone Bodies Monitored in the Original Atkins Diet

Atkins monitored carbohydrate restriction with "ketosticks." Just like the paper strips that measure glucose in the urine, these paper ketosticks measure the ketone bodies that are excreted in the urine when dietary carbohydrate is restricted.

If the diet includes fewer than 130 grams of carbohydrate, the body goes into a state of ketosis, and the diet is called a "ketogenic" diet. When carbohydrate intake falls below that level, the liver synthesizes ketone bodies that the body uses as fuel for the brain and central nervous system. Without carbohydrate in the diet, these ketone bodies provide 75% of the brain's energy. The remaining 25% comes either from glucose synthesized out of amino acids in the diet or from the breakdown of proteins in muscle tissue through a process called gluconeogenesis. A small amount also comes from glycerol that is released when triglycerides in the fat tissue are broken down into their component fatty acids.

Ketosis is a normal adaptation to a low carbohydrate diet. It should not be confused with ketoacidosis, which is a pathological state secondary to rampant diabetes. Carbohydrate-restricted diets often produce ketone levels of 5 to 20 mg/dl, which are slightly higher than levels measured after an overnight fast (5 mg/dl). Among diabetics with uncontrolled insulin levels and ketoacidosis, ketone bodies can be as high as 200 mg/dl.

Advantages and Disadvantages of the Atkin's Diet

Simply stated, the Atkins diet provides an effective way to lose weight over short periods of time (up to 3–6 months) without the side effects of food cravings and hunger attacks. The effectiveness of a high fat/protein, low carbohydrate diet was demonstrated by Blake Donaldson, Alfred Pennington, Margaret Ohlson, Charlotte Young, George Blackburn, Bruce Bistrian, Edgar Gordon, and others long before Atkins wrote *The Atkins Diet Revolution*. The success of the Atkins diet is the result of a radical reduction in carbohydrate intake, to between 60 to 130 grams (240 to 520 calories, respectively), depending on the metabolic rates of the individuals on the diet.

The main reason the Atkins diet does not work over longer periods is that few individuals can restrict their carbohydrate intake to such low levels on a continuing basis. Draconian reductions in carbohydrate are difficult to maintain without meal replacement strategies. Given the overabundance of carbohydrates in our society, carbohydrate intake invariably increases over time. When carbohydrates are unconsciously added to high fat/protein diets with unrestricted calories, the "diet" quickly turns into a regimen containing excess calories from all three food components—carbohydrate, fat, and protein—a sure prescription for rapid weight gain! Excess fat, protein, and carbohydrate combine to create the deadliest diet known to mankind.

In fact, Dr. Atkins may be one of the best arguments against the long-term use of the Atkins diet. When he died suddenly on the streets of NYC in 2004, he weighed 258 pounds. Whatever the reason for his weight gain, the lesson is clear: short-term success and safety cannot necessarily be correlated with long-term success and safety.

Comparison of Low Fat/Protein and High Fat/Protein Diets

With the exception of processed foods, fat normally follows protein in the diet. Low-fat diets are normally low in protein and high-protein diets are normally high in fat. Conversely, a diet that is low in fat and protein is normally high in carbohydrates, while a high fat/protein diet is normally low in carbohydrate.

It is therefore of great interest to compare the results of the two contrasting diets over the past 100 years, as reported by Gary Taubes. In general, diets from both groups were administered and monitored for periods of 4 months to more than 1 year.

Table 1-2

Diet	Total calories	Carb calories	Hunger	Weight loss per month
Low fat/ protein, high carbohydrate (Semi-starvation)	1,300–1,700	500–1,000	Extreme	0 – 1.5 lbs
High fat/protein, low carbohydrate (Ad libitum*)	1,500–3,000	<240	Satiation	8 – 12 lbs

*Ad libitum: At pleasure

Conclusions on Low Fat/Protein Versus High Fat/Protein Diets

Based on this analysis, we can make tentative conclusions about the efficiency with which these diets achieve successful weight loss. These conclusions may lead to hypotheses that can be tested in future studies. Fortunately, because the patterns are consistent within each individual group and the outcomes are sufficiently different between the two groups, we can draw the following tentative conclusions with some degree of certainty:

- Fat and protein diets are more satiating because fat and protein have greater effects on appetite reduction. Furthermore, fat and protein digest more slowly, leading to more pronounced feelings of satiation.
- Carbohydrate diets are less satiating because carbohydrate has less effect on reduction of hunger. Furthermore, carbohydrates, and particularly refined sugars, are rapidly digested and absorbed into the body, often leading to food swings that increase appetite.
- Weight loss and hunger are not necessarily related to the absolute number of calories consumed.
- Both satiety and weight loss are dependent on low carbohydrate levels in the diet.
- Thresholds for carbohydrate-induced weight gains vary among individual subjects.
- High-protein diets are optimal in achieving weight loss without stimulating hunger.

Under conditions of excess calories, carbohydrate in the diet appears to lead to both hunger and weight gain. In a high-fat/protein diet, excess calories may also lead to weight gain, while hunger is apparently satiated at lower levels of food consumption. During short-term dieting, it is easier to lose weight with a high fat/protein diet than it is with a low-fat/protein diet. Furthermore, it appears that weight loss with a high-fat/protein diet occurs even when a greater number of calories are consumed.

One thing seems to be certain: Not all calories are created equal. They may be equal on an energetics basis, but they are not equal on a body-weight-management basis. The long-held premise that calories are equal and therefore interchangeable between food groups in dietary management is simply not true. This subject is discussed in greater detail in chapter 9.

Hypothesis Testing

Now that we have strong hypotheses about which food groups lead to obesity, let us test these hypotheses on non-traditional diets observed in a cult society. One such cult that is known for extreme obesity is the Sumo Wrestlers in Japan. Wrestlers in this group actively seek to gain enormous weight to improve their athletic performance. While in their early twenties, their weight commonly exceeds 300 pounds.

In 1976, a team of investigators at the University of Tokyo, led by Tsuneo Nishizawa, presented a detailed study of the sumo diet, body composition, and health in the *American Journal of Clinical Nutrition*. A detailed analysis of their food intake, broken down by carbohydrate, fat, and protein and related to body fat, muscle, and athletic prowess, as shown below, is highly instructive and allows us independently to examine whether carbohydrates play a pivotal role in obesity.

Table 1-3

Nutrients	Upper Group More muscle, less fat	Lower group Less muscle, more fat
Calories	5,500	5,120
Carbohydrate	780 g (57%)	1,000g (80%)
Fat	100g (16%)	50g (9%)
Protein	365g (27%)	165g (11%)

Sumo wrestlers are divided into two groups, an "upper group" and a "lower group." Members of the upper group, who carry more muscle and less fat, represent the best wrestlers in the Japan. Members of the lower group, with less muscle and more fat, show inferior wrestling performance.

Sumo wrestlers increase their body weight by eating large quantities of Chanko Nabe, a type of pork stew, for years or even decades. Members of both groups ingest more than twice the number of calories than observed with the typical Japanese male. However, the percentage of food types differs between the two groups. Members of the upper group ingest more than twice the carbohydrates and roughly half the fat ingested by the typical Japanese person. Protein consumption is four and a half times greater than average. Compared to members of the upper group, members of the lower group ingest even greater quantities of carbohydrate while restricting relative amounts of fat and protein.

We would naturally expect that the over-abundance of calories would lead, in both cases, to extreme obesity. And it does. Nevertheless, despite their reduced fat consumption, the lower group shows significantly more fat than the upper group. It is hard to escape the conclusion that the increased carbohydrate and decreased protein content was the cause of the increased fat and poor performance of the lower group.

Summary

One of the great limitations in dietary studies is that it is impossible, by strict scientific standards, to vary a single parameter. Every change in a dietary formula involves at least two changes. For example, if you change protein in the diet and keep the amounts of fat and carbohydrate constant, you necessarily change the total amount of calories. The same is true whether you individually vary fat or carbohydrate and whether you conduct the experiment in laboratory animals or man. This conundrum explains many of the difficulties in drawing firm conclusions from any single dietary study. For example, it is not possible to determine if the effect of a high-fat/protein diet is due to the high proportion of fat and protein, low levels of carbohydrate, or both.

It is no wonder that a century of dietary studies has produced conflicting theories and recommendations. The exhaustive review by Gary

Taubes has been important for elucidating our current understanding of the mechanisms of fat storage, which significantly impacts overweight disorders and obesity.

While overweight disorders and obesity have a genetic component, changes in dietary intake can have dramatic effects on body weight. The data presented in this chapter clearly indicate that high-fat/protein diets are considerably more efficient in stimulating weight loss than low-fat/protein diets. Analysis of the results indicate that high protein/fat, low carbohydrate diets may show, on average, 5 to 10 times greater weight loss than that observed with high carbohydrate, low protein/fat diets. As such, the data provide the initial clues that carbohydrate calories are more harmful than fat calories in leading to unwanted weight gains. However, high fat/protein, low carbohydrate diets only work for a limited period of time, measured in weeks to months when carbohydrate intake is drastically reduced.

In order to understand the counterintuitive dietary and weight loss findings that have been collected over a period of more than 100 years, it is necessary to understand in, more detail, how the body regulates caloric intake, distribution, storage, and utilization of carbohydrate, fat, and protein. In Chapters 2 through 8, we will examine the scope of the problem in terms of diseases that are linked to dietary causes and will examine the scientific details that help us understand the harmful effects of carbohydrates, particularly refined sugars, on metabolic health that impacts heavily on body weight. Chapter 9 will describe the lingering paradoxes that strongly suggest there still remains a missing piece in our understanding of body weight control.

Starting in Chapter 10, we begin to reveal the missing piece as "Selective Protein Deficiency Syndrome," a newly discovered medical deficiency, which appears to cause an imbalance in metabolic pathways that control fat storage and fat metabolism. Selective protein deficiency syndrome occurs when amino acids, particularly essential and positive-charged amino acids, become deficient in our diet. A deficiency of positive-charged amino acids leads to a deficiency in positive-charged proteins that result in the imbalance in metabolic pathways. Fortunately, these deficiencies can be corrected by administering essential and positive-charged amino acids, which we define in this book as "power amino acids." The designation of "power" is used because the effects of these amino acids on body weight health are truly "powerful."

Chapter 2

Diseases of Civilization

Anthropology of Food Cultures

The disciplines of anthropology and epidemiology have shed considerable light on the historical relationships among diet, lifestyle, and health. Important studies have traced the dramatic changes in food sources as the human population has increased over time throughout the world. While most people believe that the health of human populations has steadily improved over the millennia, a close analysis of the data reveals otherwise. It has become clear that the increase of carbohydrate in the diet that resulted from the agricultural revolution has led to burgeoning increases in metabolic disorders. Collectively, these may be thought of as "diseases of civilization."

Hunters and Gatherers

For two million years before the development of agriculture, humans hunted and gathered their food. These activities dictated that the human diet would consist of large and small game, insects, scavenged meat, roots, and berries. If game was scarce, humans turned to gathering plants and insects. If gathering failed, they could resort to local water holes where large game congregated in times of continuing draught.

During this Paleolithic period of prehistory, man slowly spread from the cradle of human evolution in Africa to other parts of the world. The success of these migrations depended on the development of technologies that permitted humans to live in more extreme climates and adapt to differing food sources. 60,000 years ago, fewer than 100,000 people were estimated to be living as nomadic tribes in Africa. 40,000 years ago there were approximately 600,000 people living in Africa and, with the spread of humans to other parts of the world, 150,000 people living in Europe and West Asia.

Agriculture and Agrarian Societies

The agricultural revolution occurred during the Neolithic period, roughly 5,000 to 10,000 years ago. With the rapid development of agricultural methods, the population of Europe and Asia increased exponentially to 100 million people about 2,500 years ago and in excess of 6 billion people today.

Anthropologists who have studied human remains from before and after the agricultural revolution, from hunter-gatherers to farming communities, respectively, have concluded that nutrition and health both declined after the development of agriculture. While the reasons for this decline are not completely understood, it is believed that the rapid rise in human populations in diverse ecosystems created the need for novel food selection to maintain health. In addition, the incremental steps in the processing of foods may have improved the digestibility and color of food products. However, processing also removed protein, fiber, vitamins, minerals, and micronutrients.

At the same time, agricultural technologies led to an enormous increase in carbohydrates, initially complex carbohydrates and later refined sugars. As we will see, excessive consumption of refined and complex carbohydrates produces deleterious metabolic consequences that may result in accelerated aging and early death. The very success humans experienced in their evolution of food supplies ultimately led to conditions that compromised health.

Early Epidemiology Studies

Early studies by physicians and anthropologists in the Old World correlated changes in diets with apparent changes in the spectrum of disease and first called attention to the notion of "diseases of civilization."

As early as the late 19th century, Thomas Allinson, a physician who headed the English Bread and Food Reform League, wrote, that refined carbohydrates were a "great curse." They were responsible, he said, for the "constipation of the bowel which is caused in great measure by white bread. From this constipation come piles, varicose veins, headaches, miserable feelings, dullness and other ailments."

In the early 20th century, the physician Samuel Hutton spent 11 years on the northern coast of Labrador studying native and urbanized Eskimo populations. The native Eskimo diet was composed primarily of meat, with very few vegetables. In 1902, Hutton reported that these Eskimos appeared to be free of tumorous growths, asthma, and appendicitis. He contrasted them to Eskimos living near European settlements who consumed a diet consisting of "tea, bread, ship's biscuits, molasses and salt fish or pork." Those Eskimos who ate the "settler's dietary" were "less robust," suffered more from scurvy and fatigue, and had children who were "puny and feeble."

In 1923 after 6 years working in a native hospital in South Africa, F.P. Fouche wrote, "I never saw a single case of gastric or duodenal ulcer, colitis, appendicitis, or cancer in any form in a native although these diseases were frequently seen among the white or European population."

In their 1937 study, *Man, Bread & Destiny: The Story of Man and his Food*, C.C. Furnas and S.M. Furnas noted that, "The world is gradually going carbohydrate. That is because there are more people than there have ever been before so there must be more food. You can get about eight times as many calories from an acre of corn as you can from the flesh of pigs fed on this same corn. Because of population pressure, certain sections of the world are progressively using more of the vegetable and less of animal materials. This means that the carbohydrates from sugar and cereals particularly are increasing steadily in quantity." Furnas and Furnas went on to conclude that "this is not the best road to health," because the starches and sugars that are "low in the essentials we must have for good health," effectively replaced foods that were more important for health.

In 1967, F.T. Sai, the Regional Nutrition Officer for Africa in the Food and Agricultural Organization, commented about the rapid adoption of high-starch staples: "The potato took 200–250 years, in spite of organized encouragement, to become accepted in England. It took only fifty years in Ireland. Maize and cassava have come to be accepted in parts of Africa in considerably less time....Tea, white bread, rice and soft drinks have entered many African dietaries in even shorter time and the extent to which they have spread and their consequences to nutrition have been rather severe."

Epidemiology Studies between Native
and Urban Societies in the Old World

Epidemiology studies in societies that have been transported from native environments to urban environments have been particularly helpful in linking differences in the patterns of human disease to differences in diet.

Yemenite Jews

Since the 1930s, a population of urban Jews from Yemen lived in Israel. A new group of Yemeni Jews was flown into Israel in 1949 as part of "Operation Magic Carpet" shortly after the state of Israel was founded. The incidence of diabetes, heart disease, hypertension, and high cholesterol levels was far greater in the group that had been in Israel since the 1930s than in the later immigrant group. Yet, the only significant difference between the two populations of Yemeni Jews was in the consumption of processed sugar, which was significantly higher in the former group.

New Zealand Maoris

Cardiologist Ian Prior studied the Maoris living in New Zealand. Converted to the civilized diet of New Zealand, these native tribes had a higher incidence of diabetes, heart disease, obesity, and gout. Sixty percent of the middle-aged women were overweight. Over one third were obese. Sixteen percent had heart disease. Six percent of the men had diabetes. The diets of the Maori in NZ were bread, flour, biscuits, breakfast cereals, sugar (greater than 70 pound per person per year), and potatoes. There was also an abundance of beer, ice cream, soft drinks, and sweets. Tea was the common beverage, "taken with large amounts of sugar by the majority."

Indian Migrants in South Africa

In the 1950s, George Campbell studied two populations of Indian immigrants living in the Natal region of South Africa. Natal Indians were brought to South Africa in the latter half of the 19th century to work as indentured laborers on the local sugar plantations. Seventy percent were impoverished and many still worked for the sugar plantations. All sugar cane workers were given a weekly ration of 1.5 pounds of sugar. Furthermore, by chewing sugar cane they could augment their intake by

0.5 to 1.0 pound daily! Out of a local population of 250,000, Campbell's clinic treated 6,200 for diabetes.

Natal Indians were compared to rural Zulus, another group of Indian immigrants who were living under native conditions. The per capita consumption of sugar for rural Zulus was similar to those living in India, around 12 pounds yearly, compared with nearly 80 pounds for working-class Natal Indians. The peak incubation period of diabetes for the Natal Indians lay between 18 and 22 years.

Natal Indians showed similar diseases to local whites, who suffered from diabetes, coronary thrombosis, hypertension, appendicitis, gall bladder disease, and other diseases of civilization. The rural Zulus had none of these diseases. Despite thousands of exams, diabetes has never been diagnosed in the native population.

Later, Dr. Campbell spent a year working at the Hospital of the University of Pennsylvania in Philadelphia and was astonished by the similarity of the black population in Philadelphia to his white patients in Durban, South Africa, and the complete dissimilarity with the black population of rural Zulus.

In 1966, Campbell joined with Thomas Cleave, a surgeon in the British Royal Navy, to publish *Diabetes, Coronary Thrombosis and the Saccharine Disease.* Campbell and Cleave argued that *all* the significant chronic diseases of civilization were caused by sugar and by starch, which the body converts to sugar. These disorders included not just diabetes and heart disease, but a wide spectrum of disorders, including obesity, peptic ulcers, and appendicitis. Taken as a group, they were called "refined carbohydrate diseases."

The Pima Indians in the New World
For a long time, the Pima Indians of Arizona have suffered from obesity. Today, they have the highest documented rates of obesity and diabetes in the United States—up to 82%. This tribe of Indians has been the focus of repeated studies by the National Institutes of Health over the past 50 years. In fact, they are among the most studied groups of people in the world.

For 2,000 years, the Pima lived as hunters and gatherers. They had ample access to game and fish, and by the time Jesuit missionaries arrived in last half of the eighteenth century, the tribe had already learned to harvest corn and beans on irrigated fields. Over the ensuing decades, they continued to develop into an agrarian society. In 1846, a U.S. army observer passed through Pima lands and declared that the Pima were "sprightly" and in "fine health."

When the California gold rush opened a wagon route through Pima territory, it brought people and civilization from around the world to the Pima villages. At first, these travelers bought food and supplies from the Pima as they made their way to the gold country. By the 1860s, this traffic had slowed, and the Anglo-Americans and Mexicans who came to Pima territory were more likely to settle. These settlers changed the life of the Pima Indians forever. They hunted the game the Pima had depended on and appropriated the water for their own settlements. Before the century had ended, the Pima had endured "years of famine" so severe that they became dependent on government handouts of foodstuffs. At the same time, they became obese to a degree unparalleled among other American Indian tribes.

By 1905 the Pima diet included, in the words of Aleš Hrdlička[1] , "everything…that enters into the dietary of the white man." This included "sugar, coffee, and canned foods to replace traditional foodstuffs lost ever since whites had settled in their territories." It has been estimated that 50% of their calories came from sugar and flour.

By the 1950s, obesity and poverty were connected once again when the anthropologist Bertram Kraus noted the troubling fact that half the Pima children on the reservation were obese before they were 11 years old. Subsequent studies into their diet documented the alarming proportion of calories that came from carbohydrates and processed foods. By 1973, the epidemiologist Peter Bennett told George McGovern's Senate Committee on Nutrition and Human Needs that half of all Pima were diabetic because of the amount of sugar in their diet. "The only question that I would have," Bennett said, "is whether we can implicate sugar specifically or whether the important factor is not calories in general, which in fact turns out to be really excessive amounts of carbohydrates." This opinion was reinforced 16 years later by Henry Dobyns, who reported that "many of the poorer individuals subsist on a diet of potatoes, bread, and other starchy foods."

Other Indians

The diet of the Pima Indians is consistent with the diet of numerous Indian tribes that have been relegated to government-supported reservations, including the Sioux of the South Dakota's Crow Creek Reservation, the Arizona Apaches, the North Carolina Cherokees, and all the Oklahoma tribes. All of these Indian tribes also display levels of obesity comparable to the Pima Indians living in poverty today.

For example, the staple on the Sioux reservation is something called "grease bread," which is made from white flour and fried in fat. Grease Bread is often combined with high-carbohydrate foods like oatmeal, potatoes, beans, squash, canned tomatoes, canned milk, and sugar, all fried together into a kind of omelet. The men are fat, and the women are fatter.

The salient point is that Indians living in poverty and suffering from obesity consume diets that are carbohydrate-rich and protein-poor. These patterns are observed not only among groups in the United States, but also among impoverished groups in Africa and the West Indies, who ingest carbohydrate-rich diets that are long on refined sugar and short on protein.

Diseases of Civilization

It is patently clear from these anthropological and epidemiological studies that diabetes, obesity, coronary heart disease, gallstones, gall bladder disease, cavities, and periodontal disease are linked to the dietary effects of civilization. Cleave and Campbell reported that the primary change in traditional diets following westernization has been the addition of sugar, flour, and white rice and that these dietary changes occurred shortly before the appearance of the chronic diseases.

According to Cleave, the processing of refined sugars leads to damage in three ways:

- Overconsumption of calories: A teaspoon of sugar contains as many calories as an apple. However, individuals easily eat many teaspoons of sugar. By contrast, an individual can eat only one or two apples.
- Removal of protein in the refining process: Proteins are often stripped away from foods during the refining process. This typically increases the relative proportion of calories that come from carbohydrates and reduces the proportion of calories from protein.
- An increase in the rate of carbohydrate absorption: The refining process increases the rate of absorption of sugars into the blood stream.

For example, the sugar contained in the starch of a potato is absorbed more slowly than concentrated sugar because starch requires digestion to break the carbohydrate into sugar building blocks. Starch contains linear and branched chains of sugars that may be 10,000 units long. In contrast, sucrose (cane sugar) contains disaccharides, two sugar units consisting of glucose and fructose.

John Yudkin and Sugar

In 1953, John Yudkin founded the Department of Nutrition at Queen Elizabeth College in London. A few years later, he wrote *The Slimming Business,* in which he advocated a very low carbohydrate diet for weight loss.

Yudkin then studied the effects of sugar and starch fed to rats, mice, chickens, rabbits, and pigs. In varying degrees, the sugar raised cholesterol, triglycerides, and insulin levels in each of his tests. Yudkin also studied the effects of high-sugar diets on college students. He observed that their cholesterol levels, triglycerides, and insulin levels all rose, while their blood became more viscous, making the students, he thought, more susceptible to atherosclerosis and coronary heart disease.

Shortly after he retired in 1971, Yudkin outlined his sugar theory in *Sweet and Dangerous.* He argued that sugars and starches brought little of nutritional value to the diet except calories, and sugars were the worst offenders. Yudkin concluded that sugars were the first things that needed to be removed from the diet of overweight individuals.

Yudkin was discredited and ridiculed by the medical establishment, which persisted in repudiating any challenges to its orthodox position. According to Gary Taubes, those who cited Yudkin favorably were not just ignored; they were black-balled with the comment, "He's just like Yudkin."

Problems with Dietary Association Studies

In the past, epidemiologists compared the carbohydrate, protein, and fat contents of diets in different countries with mortality from various diseases. Carbohydrates were not separated into complex and refined carbohydrates (starch versus sugars). Fat was not separated into animal, vegetable, and trans (hydrogenated) fat. Intake of essential fatty acids (omega-3 and omega-6 fatty acids) was not reported. Cholesterol was not separated into LDL (bad cholesterol) and HDL (good cholesterol).

It would not be until the 1990s that the epidemiologists would begin to distinguish between complex and simple sugars and saturated and unsaturated fats in their dietary analyses.

The Role of Refined Carbohydrates

The greatest single change in the American diet over the past 200 years has been the dramatic increase in sugar consumption from the mid-nineteenth century forward. The dramatic rise is summarized in the table below:

Table 2-1

Year	Pounds of sugar consumed[1]
1830	15 lbs
1920	100 pounds
2000	150 pounds[1]

[1]includes high fructose corn syrup

Based on anthropology and epidemiology, refined sugars appear to be responsible for most of the diseases of civilization. Consider that:

- The six-country study of Ancel Keys correlated disease more with per capita consumption of sugar than with cholesterol or fat consumption
- Walter Mertz, past chairman of the USDA human Nutrition Institute, testified that refined sugars disrupt the health of laboratory animals by elevating blood sugar and triglycerides, leading to diabetes and premature death
- The beneficial effect of the Mediterranean diet may also be explained by the lack of sugar and white flour as much as the fish, olive oil, and vegetables

Cancer Linked to Diseases of Civilization

In a 16-year study of 900,000 patients reported in the *New England Journal of Medicine*, overweight males showed an increased risk of dying from prostate and colorectal cancer by 52%. Overweight women showed a 62% increase in the risk of dying from breast and pancreatic cancer. Furthermore, the risk of dying from cancer showed a linear relationship with weight increase. Women weighing 165, 200, and 245 pounds showed an 8%, 23% and 62% higher risk of dying from cancer, respectively. In men, increases in obesity led to a linear increase in dying from cancer up to 52%.

In 1975, Richard Doll and Bruce Armstrong published their seminal studies on diet and cancer. In these studies, they called attention to the strong correlation between higher sugar intake in different countries and the higher incidence of mortality from cancer of the colon, rectum, breast, ovary, uterus, and prostate.

Summary

Throughout the 20th century, epidemiological studies continued to link the dietary changes of civilized nations with the occurrence of numerous diseases not observed in primitive societies. Yet even the most compelling evidence largely fell on deaf ears in the medical establishment. Medicine paid little attention to nutrition. The idea that simple changes in diet, involving the refinement of sugar, white flour, and rice, could account for serious diseases seemed preposterous.

Yet, as we will see in later chapters, the molecular biology studies conducted over the past 50 years have led us to recognize the existence of a Metabolic Syndrome that is associated with a number of age- and death-related risk factors, including obesity, type 2 diabetes, high blood pressure, high cholesterol levels, high triglyceride levels, and increased levels of body inflammation that lead to atherosclerotic disease, heart attack and stroke. The spectrum of diseases associated with the Metabolic Syndrome, described in chapter 9, closely mimics the collection of diseases identified, in this chapter, as "diseases of civilization."

The anthropological and epidemiological studies presented here provide the initial clues that carbohydrate-rich foods and refined sugars are responsible, in part, for many of the diseases of civilization that are not observed in primitive cultures.

The more we work in the laboratory, the more we are able to identify the molecular mechanisms that produce heart disease, cancer, and the metabolic diseases that lead to early death. The role of nutritional factors in the development of these diseases is becoming increasingly clear. While dietary mechanisms do not diminish the role of genetic traits and predispositions to these diseases, it is impressive how much dietary factors appear to influence the incidence of these diseases.

In hindsight, it appears that the early observations on the associations between dietary changes and deadly disease were correct all along.

Part 2

Adaptive Change
and Energy Pathways

"The true scientist is one whose work includes both experimental theory and experimental practice. He notes a fact. A propos of this fact, an idea is born in his mind. In the light of this idea, he reasons, devises an experiment, imagines and brings to pass its material conditions. From this experiment new phenomena result which must be observed, and so on and so forth."

–Claude Bernard

Chapter 3

Adaptation of the Body to Changing Diets

Claude Bernard, the famous French physiologist who worked in the mid to late 19th century, discovered that food delivered to the small intestine stimulated the pancreas to secrete juice into the intestinal tract, where it could facilitate the absorption of food components in the diet. Later in the century, Ivan Pavlov, the Russian physiologist, discovered that the pancreatic juice contained "ferments" (later known as enzymes) that digested foods so that they could be absorbed into the body and distributed to organs and tissues via the bloodstream.

Pavlov made another significant discovery with his famous dogs by showing that the enzyme ferment in pancreatic juice could be altered by changing the food components in the diet. When dogs were fed high-protein diets consisting entirely of meat, the capacity of the pancreatic juice to digest protein increased dramatically. In contrast, when dogs were fed carbohydrate diets consisting entirely of bread, the ability of the pancreatic juice to digest carbohydrate increased dramatically. This was the first demonstration that the body could adapt to changes in the environment, in this case the composition of food in the diet (dietary adaptation is discussed in greater detail later in this chapter). It was an enormous breakthrough that helped Pavlov win the Nobel Prize.

Enzymes as the Working Units in the Body

The work of Bernard and Pavlov stimulated enormous research in the early twentieth century throughout Europe and the United States. This research identified the pancreatic enzymes that digest protein, carbohydrate, and fat in the diet. This early research on pancreatic enzymes not only became the model for later work on enzymes throughout the body; it also called attention to the essential nature of the proteins that work as enzymes to build (synthesize) and destroy (digest) structural units (proteins) in the body. This work, in turn, showed that the body was rebuilding itself on a minute-by-minute schedule, day after day, week after week, to repair cells and maintain health. The importance of body repair and health maintenance will be discussed in greater detail in chapter 11.

This research underscored the importance of diet for the health of all biological organisms, including human beings. Even today, most people do not understand or appreciate the importance of dietary renewal and repair in human health and aging.

Burst of Scientific Research in the Late Twentieth Century

In the late 1950s Congress, established the National Institutes of Health (NIH) in Bethesda, MD. It created extensive laboratories built for NIH's internal use (its intramural program), and it also funded an extramural program to provide resources for individual research projects in universities, medical schools, and hospitals throughout the United States. Congress understood that the enormous research efforts around the country would require massive financial assistance. Because these efforts shared the goal of conquering disease, the number of institutes within the NIH increased in number to reflect the expanding areas of disease focus.

As a result, the budget for the extramural programs grew from year to year until it now amounts to approximately 35 billion dollars annually. For the first time in the history of mankind, enormous efforts can be directed at understanding the molecular mechanisms of disease and the potential for curing those diseases. The expanding NIH budget allows the United States to excel in its leadership role of fighting disease not only in America but also throughout the world. The financial commitment to biological research in this country is enormous. The NIH budget is now 40 times the budget for medical research in the UK, which ranks second among national research funding throughout the world.

Much of what we know today about management of human disease, including the impressive advances in diagnostic tests and treatment protocols, is the result of the enormous financial commitments of the NIH. Among the many achievements of NIH-sponsored research in every field of medicine, perhaps the greatest accomplishment was the Human Genome Project, which successfully sequenced the 3 billion pairs of nucleotides (the human genome) that form the DNA archive that houses the estimated 20,000 genes that reside on 23 chromosomes in the human body. America has benefited immeasurably from the resulting advances in science and medicine, and the world has benefited as well. Much of the material presented in the rest of this book relies on information supported by the National Institutes of Health.

2D Gel Electrophoresis and the Proteome of Digestive Enzymes

In 1975, I invented a technique called two-dimensional gel electrophoresis, which revolutionized the separation of complex mixtures of proteins throughout the human body. I was a young scientist working at the Rockefeller University where, with research support from the NIH, I developed this technique for separating proteins in higher animals, including mammals and humans, according to their two basic physical parameters: "charge" in the first dimension and "size" in the second dimension.[1] The 2D gel allowed researchers for the first time to make detailed analyses of the complete repertoire of proteins in organs, tissues, and body fluids. Over time, "protein profiles" have contributed to our understanding of the sum total of all the proteins in the human body, which contains approximately 20,000 distinct proteins. This inventory of proteins with diverse functions is known as the Human Proteome. It includes proteins from all of the organs and tissues throughout the body. The 2D gel electrophoresis technique is now used in all of the major medical research institutions around the world.

This breakthrough allowed my laboratory, which focused on digestive enzymes (proteins) contained in pancreatic tissues and secretions, to make a number of seminal observations in the field of biological adaptation, a field that was poorly understood in the early 1970s. Nutritional scientists who had previously investigated biological adaptation in proteins to changes in dietary composition had been unable to discover changes in protein profiles. For example, measurements of protein in blood or tissues were conducted on either total protein or broad subcategories of proteins (albumin and globulins). The older protein tests were incapable of providing the level of detail necessary to determine the patterns of change that caused biological adaptation or disease.

Once the 2D gel was developed, researchers could separate complex mixtures of proteins into individual forms. Thereafter, the study of biological adaptation accelerated markedly. Since most adaptation processes involved "turning on" one group of genes and their protein counterparts and "turning off" another group of genes and their protein counterparts, any technology that measured only total protein or even large subgroups of proteins would not have the resolution to detect important changes at the level of individual proteins. They would often miss the global changes as well.

As soon as we applied the 2D gel to the analysis of dietary adaptation in the pancreas, we quickly observed the patterns of response. We first isolated and analyzed all sixteen digestive enzymes produced by the pancreas in several species (see Appendix). Figure 1 shows human pancreatic digestive enzymes separated in a 2D gel; it demonstrates the ease with which these proteins can be separated. Table 1 lists these proteins according to name, function, and their two basic physical parameters, "charge," and "size."

Figure 3-1: 2D Gel of human pancreatic digestive enzymes

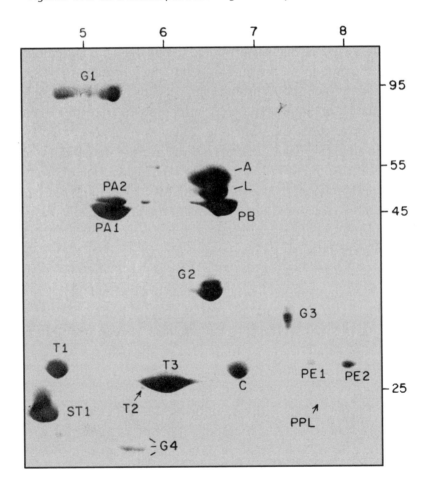

Table 3-1: protein characteristics

	I.U.B. Number	Abbrev.	$M_r{}^a$	$IEP_n{}^b$	$IEP_u{}^c$	Mass proportion (%)^d	Distribution of stain (%)^e	PAS^f
1. Glycoprotein 1		G1	93,000	3.9	5.0	3.1	7.5	+
2. α-Amylase	(EC 3.2.1.1)	A	54,800	6.3	6.4	5.3	18.3	−
3. Lipase	(EC 3.1.1.3)	L	50,500	6.5	6.6	0.7	3.0	+
4. (Pro)carboxypeptidase A1	(EC 3.4.17.1)	PA1	46,000	4.6	5.1	16.8	12.9	−
5. (Pro)carboxypeptidase A2	(EC 3.4.17.1)	PA2	47,000	4.7	5.5	8.1	1.2	−
6. (Pro)carboxypeptidase B1	(EC 3.4.17.2)	PB1	47,000	6.2	6.7	4.4	8.2	−
7. (Pro)carboxypeptidase B2	(EC 3.4.17.2)	PB2	47,000	6.7	6.8	2.9	—	−
8. Glycoprotein 2		G2	36,500	5.2	6.6	6.7	8.1	+
9. Glycoprotein 3^g		G3	—	7.2	7.0	0.5	1.7	+
10. Trypsin(ogen) 1	(EC 3.4.21.4)	T1	28,000	4.4	4.9	23.1	9.3	−
11. Trypsin(ogen) 2	(EC 3.4.21.4)	T2	26,000	5.5	5.7	—	—	−
12. Trypsin(ogen) 3	(EC 3.4.21.4)	T3	26,700	6.4	6.2	16.0	18.1	−
13. Chymotrypsin(ogen)	(EC 3.4.21.1)	C	29,000	7.2	6.8	1.7	7.0	−
14. (Pro)elastase 1	(EC 3.4.21.11)	PE1	30,500	7.6	7.2	3.1	1.0	−
15. (Pro)elastase 2	(EC 3.4.21.11)	PE2	30,500	>7.9	8.0	1.2	1.3	−
16. Glycoprotein 4		G4	15,700	5.4	5.5	2.5	1.1	+
17. Colipase 1		CL1	—	7.2	7.3	—	—	−
18. Colipase 2		CL2	—	7.4	7.4	—	—	−
19. (Pro)phospholipase A$_2$	(EC 3.1.1.4)	PPL	17,500	7.5	7.9	—	—	−

After we identified the complete inventory of digestive enzymes (the digestive proteome), we determined all the adaptations in digestive enzyme profiles that resulted from changes in protein, carbohydrate, and fat in the diet. When diets were rich in carbohydrate, we saw increases in carbohydrate-digesting enzymes (amylases). We saw increases in fat-digesting enzymes (lipases) when diets were rich in fat and increases in protein-digesting enzymes (proteases or proteinases) when diets were rich in protein.

These results allowed us to discover the "purposeful" feedback mechanisms that govern dietary adaptation patterns. When carbohydrate levels in the diet increase, the pancreas adapts by increasing the production of amylases. When protein levels increase in the diet, the pancreas increases the production of proteases and decreases the production of amylases. We saw the same phenomenon when increased levels of fat in the diet led to increased production of lipases and decreased production of amylases and proteases.[2]

Hormones Regulate Adaptation Pathways

Next, we discovered the mechanisms by which the body provides this purposeful feedback regulation. Each feedback mechanism depends on specific hormones. The hormone cholecystokinin (CCK) is responsible for the feedback that "tells" the pancreas to increase the production of proteases when dietary protein increases. The hormone secretin stimulates the pancreas to produce increased lipases when fats increase in the diet. And the hormone insulin triggers the pancreas to produce more amylases when the carbohydrate increases. The results are summarized in the following table.

Table 3-2

Dietary components	Digestive end products	Hormone regulators	Digestive Enzymes		
			Proteinases	Lipases	Amylases
Protein	Amino acids	CCK	Increased		
Fat	Fatty acids	Secretin		Increased	
Carbs	Glucose	Insulin			Increased

These findings show the remarkable ability of the human body to adapt to changes in food components in the diet. They also demonstrate that the adaptation is not a random event, as discussed earlier in this chapter. Selective feedback mechanisms that operate through specific hormone-receptor interactions and stimulus-response coupling enable the body to shift from one digestive pattern to another as the composition of the diet changes.

Disruption in Adaptive Pathways

These studies also show that adaptation of the body to changing environmental conditions is one of the fundamental laws of human biology. The body smoothly adapts from one dietary pattern to another, and the purposefully adaptive patterns increase the efficiency with which the body extracts the maximal number of calories in changing diets. These metabolic efficiencies serve the body well when food is scarce in the environment. They help promote survival in primitive circumstances.

However, in today's world of overabundant food, these efficiencies may promote metabolic reactions that lead to suffering and disease. We will see later that dietary adaptation functions smoothly only when adequate amounts of protein are maintained in the diet. Under conditions of protein deficiency, serious disruptions occur in the feedback mechanisms that regulate pancreatic adaptations to changing diets. The disruptions caused by protein deficiency may, in fact, be so severe that they threaten the basic mechanisms of human health. One of these disruptions is the promotion of overweight disorders and obesity. And these disruptions may lead to the diseases of civilization that accelerate aging as well.

Summary

The burst of scientific research in the late 20th century in the United States led the way to scientific discoveries that have elucidated the molecular mechanisms of human health and disease. Impressive progress has been made in understanding how organs and tissues throughout the body adapt to changes in the environment, including changes in specific nutrients in the diet.

Studies on the exocrine pancreas, which produces the majority of enzymes involved in food digestion, led the way to understanding how the pancreas adapts to changes in the diet. These studies were greatly facilitated by the invention of 2D gel electrophoresis which allowed my laboratory to study the synthesis, transport and secretion of the complete repertoire of pancreatic enzymes into the intestinal tract where digestive processes take place.

Pancreatic adaptation allows the body to adjust to changes in food substrates (protein, carbohydrate and fat) in the diet by changing the mixture of enzymes that are released into the intestine. These adaptive changes are "purposeful," meaning that the body provides the right mixture of enzymes to digest the constituents found in the diet. As such adaptation is one of the fundamental laws of human biology.

Further studies revealed the hormones that regulate these adaptation pathways, which ensure the overall nutritional health of the body. Within limits, the body is capable of adjusting or adapting seamlessly to the changes in dietary composition. However, beyond certain limits, disruptions occur in these adaptive pathways that have the potential to lead to disease states, including selective protein deficiency syndrome and metabolic disorders that may lead to chronic degenerative diseases and obesity, as discussed in the later chapters of this book.

However, we need to first understand the energy pathways in the body and how these pathways are regulated by hormones to distribute fat and carbohydrate throughout the body.

Chapter 4

Energy Pathways within the Body

The body contains separate and distinct energy pathways that convert the three types of food in the diet into energy the body can use. Each of the substrates—protein, fat, and carbohydrate—is continuously being broken down and resynthesized. The body evolved these dynamic processes to ensure that the structural units of life remain functional in the face of numerous non-specific processes, such as environmental factors that modify and destroy these important elements.

Nothing in the body is static. Under conditions of changing patterns in food availability, the body evolved intricate mechanisms to shift energy pathways from one food type to another. While energy may be utilized from protein, fat, and carbohydrate, the main shifts in energy pathways involve inverse processes of carbohydrate and fat metabolism. When blood sugar and insulin are high, feedback mechanisms inhibit fat utilization. In contrast, when blood sugar and insulin levels are low, feedback mechanisms promote fat utilization. The broad scope of these inverse changes in energy utilization has been referred to as "fuel partitioning."

A complete understanding of the mechanisms of fuel partitioning provides the secrets to weight control in today's society.

Energy Utilization from Protein Metabolism

During their hunter-gatherer history, humans regulated energy metabolism mainly by regulating protein and fat intake. The human food chain was largely built at the top of a process in which larger animals fed off smaller animals. In the beginning, the primary food source was game. Meat ingested from game consisted mainly of protein and fat.

In many ways, protein represents the best source of nutrition and energy. It is totally self-sufficient, in that protein by itself supports the entirety of life. The same cannot be said for carbohydrate or fat.

Protein not only provides amino acids, the building blocks of life, but it also acts as a source of energy for metabolism. Protein can also be converted into sugars through a process called gluconeogenesis. Through a fundamental process called the Krebs cycle, protein can also give rise to the production of lipids and fats that are important for cellular membranes.

Krebs Cycle and Energy Production

In the 1930s, Hans Krebs documented the metabolic pathways[1] that convert nutrients delivered through the blood stream into usable energy within cells. Dependent on a process called oxidative phosphorylation, these metabolic operations are performed in mitochondria[2] to convert the fat, carbohydrate, and protein into adenosine triphosphate (ATP), which serves as a short-term energy intermediate.

Following its creation in mitochondria, ATP is transported into the cell cytoplasm, where it serves as an energy source for enzymatic reactions. When ATP gives up a phosphate molecule to become adenosine diphosphate (ADP), it releases the energy that is necessary for enzyme activity to have its beneficial effects. It is not surprising that enzymes, often described as the "working units" of the cell, require energy to function as modifiers of molecular structures through synthetic (constructive) or hydrolytic (digestive) reactions.

The Krebs Cycle conclusively demonstrates how the body can switch from one energy pathway to another and still provide ATP for energy-requiring enzymatic reactions within cells.

Energy Utilization from Fat Metabolism

In the natural food chain, protein is usually associated with copious amounts of fat. As hunters and gatherers, our forbearers developed highly efficient systems for absorbing, distributing, storing, and utilizing fat. Fat in the diet is first transported by the portal circulation from the intestinal tract to the liver, where it is processed into lipoprotein particles for delivery throughout the body. Within the liver, carbohydrates may also be converted into triglycerides by a process known as *de novo lipogenesis* and then packaged into lipoprotein particles that are distributed in the same manner.

While fat is stored in cells and transferred in the blood circulation as triglycerides, it passes across membranes as free fatty acids. Elaborate enzymatic systems have evolved in multiple sites throughout the body to breakdown triglycerides into their component parts, including free fatty acids and glycerol phosphate (lipolysis), and to re-synthesize triglycerides (fat) from the same free fatty acids and glycerol phosphate (lipogenesis). Both processes occur simultaneously inside fat cells as part of a dynamic process known as the triglyceride/fatty acid cycle.

Edgar Gordon, the endocrinologist from the University of Wisconsin, stated in 1969 that "The storage of triglyceride fat in widely scattered adipose tissue sites is a remarkably dynamic process, with the stream of fatty acid carbon atoms flowing in widely fluctuating amounts, first in one direction and then the other in a finely adjusted minute by minute response to the fuel requirements of energy metabolism in the whole organism." The American Physiological Society's 1965 *Handbook of Physiology*, stated, a "ceaseless stream of [free fatty acids flow] into the bloodstream" to provide abundant energy throughout the body.

Role of Glycerol Phosphate

Free fatty acids alone are insufficient to produce triglycerides and fat tissue. A three-carbon molecule, glycerol phosphate, provides the backbone of the triglyceride unit by linking the three fatty acids together. Glycerol comes from the metabolism of carbohydrates and is essential for storing triglycerides in fat tissue.

The more glucose that is transported into the liver and fat cells—a process that depends on insulin—the more triglyceride synthesis occurs in the liver, the more lipoprotein particles are shuttled to fat depots, and the more triglycerides are stored in those depots.

When glycerol phosphate levels drop in the absence of blood glucose and insulin, the metabolic pathways shift from fat storing to fat releasing and fat burning processes.

Energy Utilization from Carbohydrate Metabolism

Early man also foraged, largely on a seasonal basis, for fruits and vegetables that are rich in complex carbohydrates. But man (and other organisms) never really ate a balanced diet. Rather, man's diet was shaped by the available food—protein and fat from game and carbohydrate from fruits and vegetables. The sources of food varied according to the season and the availability of food (animal versus plant sources). In response to these changing conditions, biological systems developed regulatory systems that allowed the body's metabolism to adapt to changing food types. Adaptation allowed homeostasis[3] and health to be maintained in spite of constantly changing environmental conditions.

As we learned in Chapter 3, specific hormones allow the body to adapt to changing conditions of food types and digestive needs, as well as changes in energy needs, changes in reproduction, changes in stress, and numerous other changes that occur in biological organisms. Under necessity to regulate the energy pathways linked to varying food sources, the body evolved hormonal mechanisms that trigger shifts from carbohydrate to fat metabolism in times of game abundance and from fat to carbohydrate metabolism in times of food abundance from fruit and vegetables.

The most important regulator between energy sources (carbohydrate versus fat/protein) is the hormone insulin. In response to intake of carbohydrate, the level of glucose increases in the bloodstream. Rises in blood glucose stimulate the pancreas to secrete greater quantities of insulin. Insulin then acts on peripheral tissues to promote the cellular absorption of glucose. Once inside cells, glucose is metabolized through the Krebs cycle and related pathways to allow the body to use glucose as its main source of energy.

However, as Solomon Berson and Rosalyn Yalow stated in the early 1960s, insulin is also "the principal regulator of fat metabolism." When insulin secretion increases into the bloodstream, glucose metabolism is stimulated and fat metabolism is reduced. When insulin secretion into the blood stream is reduced, the reverse happens. Metabolism of fat is stimulated and metabolism of carbohydrate is reduced. As metabolic pathways are regulated by insulin, the pathways for energy utilization are similarly regulated. Under conditions of high blood sugar and insulin, the body's cells will convert glucose into energy. Under conditions of low blood sugar and insulin, the body's cells will derive energy from fatty acids.

The Randle Cycle and Glucose

While glucose and fatty acid metabolism can be regulated inversely to one another, minimal glucose levels need to be maintained in the bloodstream. The body accomplishes this through the glucose/fatty acid cycle, also known as the Randle Cycle that takes its name from the British biochemist, Sir Philip Randle. When the body is primarily utilizing fatty acids as fuel, a series of reactions in muscle cells inhibit the use of glucose for fuel and substitute fatty acids instead. Despite the metabolism of fatty acid, blood glucose levels remain stabilized.

In the alternative energy state, when blood sugar is increased and insulin levels rise, cells compensate by burning more glucose, and this serves to dampen the rise in glucose levels. The Randle Cycle modulates the glucose levels in the bloodstream and keeps them from becoming too high or too low. By maintaining minimal glucose levels in the bloodstream, the organism avoids the deleterious effects of hypoglycemic and hyperglycemic reactions.

Energy Storage and Backup Systems

The human body has also evolved backup systems to store reservoirs of energy. Nearly everyone understands that fat deposits provide long-term energy stores. Fat storage enables the body to meet its energy needs over periods of days to months.

Long distance runners are aware that the liver and muscle tissues store glycogen as a short-term source of carbohydrate energy. Carbohydrate storage mechanisms meet energy needs over periods of minutes to hours. Divergent energy needs and storage mechanisms explain why fat storage systems are more efficient (9 calories of energy are released from 1 gram of fat) than carbohydrate storage systems (4 calories of energy are released from 1 gram of carbohydrate). For the same reason, the body is able to store much more energy as fat than it is able to store carbohydrate energy in the form of glycogen.

The purpose of this book is to show that dietary habits can be changed to optimize energy storage and use and to minimize excessive fat stores. Understanding how the body manages caloric intake and shifts energy pathways from carbohydrate to fat provides the foundation for understanding how to maintain optimal body weight and fat tissue.

Summary

While the pathways for storage and utilization of protein, fat, and carbohydrate in the body are separate and distinct, the metabolites from each of these energy pathways are ultimately processed by the Krebs cycle in the mitochondria. Fuel substrates are converted from the divergent sources into energy as adenosine triphosphate (ATP), which fuels the cellular enzymes that are essential for health and life.

The body has developed intricate systems for storage of protein in muscle, carbohydrate as glycogen in liver and fat as triglycerides in adipose tissue. The pathways for utilization of substrates is called fuel partitioning and hormones regulate fuel partitioning between carbohydrate and fat storage sites.

A complete understanding of the mechanisms of fuel partitioning provides the secrets to weight control in today's society. The next four chapters focus on understanding these energy pathways in greater detail.

Chapter 5

Hormones Regulate
Energy Pathways and Appetite

Insulin

In 1960, Rosalyn Yalow and Solomon Berson developed the first accurate and reliable method for measuring the concentration of insulin and other peptide hormones in the bloodstream. This was a revolutionary development, since peptide hormones are present in the bloodstream only in minute concentrations. For her breakthrough discoveries, Yalow won the Nobel Prize in 1977 (Berson had died in 1972).

The discovery of reliable methods to measure peptide hormones in blood turned the world of diabetes on its head. Yalow and Berson showed that circulating insulin levels were significantly higher in adults who suffered from adult-onset diabetes than in healthy individuals. In 1965, they showed that not only did these diabetics have an excess of insulin in the blood, but their tissues also did not respond properly to the insulin they secreted. In addition to being hyperglycemic, with high blood glucose, and hyperinsulemic, with high blood insulin, they were *insulin resistant*.

These findings revolutionized our understanding of diabetes. It had long been assumed that all forms of diabetes were caused by a lack of insulin. This breakthrough underscored the fact that diabetes occurred in two distinct forms. Type I diabetes, also known as childhood diabetes, was the result of an inability of beta cells in the pancreas to produce insulin. Type II diabetes, also known as adult-onset diabetes, was due to insulin resistance.

These discoveries about insulin also paved the road to a new understanding of diet and obesity. By the mid 1970s, breakthroughs in hormone measurements reinforced the finding that insulin levels regulate energy shifts between carbohydrate metabolism and fat metabolism.

Insulin Shifts Energy Utilization Pathways

Insulin is the most powerful regulator of energy metabolism. It therefore serves as the body's primary *energy switch*. When blood glucose increases, corresponding insulin increases promote glucose metabolism and stimulate metabolic processes that burn sugar. At the same time insulin blocks fat metabolism.

However, when blood-glucose levels decrease, as typically occurs in between meals, insulin levels drop and metabolic processes that burn sugar become inhibited. Low insulin levels stimulate the release of fatty acids from fat depots. Blood levels of triglycerides increase, and cells and tissues switch to energy pathways that utilize free fatty acids.

Insulin Stimulates Carbohydrate Metabolism

As the master energy switch, insulin switches energy utilization from triglyceride pathways (fat metabolism) to sugar pathways (carbohydrate metabolism). In other words, carbohydrates stimulate insulin secretion, and insulin shifts fat-burning pathways to carbohydrate-burning pathways. As a consequence, increases in blood sugar (hyperglycemia) and insulin levels (hyperinsulinemia) act together to stimulate carbohydrate metabolism.

Insulin Increases Fat Storage and Accumulation

As a consequence of insulin's action as the master switch in energy pathways, increases in blood sugar (hyperglycemia) and insulin levels (hyperinsulinemia) act together to block fat metabolism. As a result, insulin is also responsible for stimulating fat accumulation by depositing calories as fat and inhibiting the utilization of fat for fuel. Because of the behavior of insulin, therefore, *dietary carbohydrates promote excess fat accumulation.*

Insulin is such a powerful energy switch that it is the *only* hormone to promote fat accumulation. Thus, it is likely to play an important role in overweight disorders and obesity. It follows that metabolic strategies to reduce stores of fat in the body must pay attention to carbohydrate intake and insulin elevations.

Biological Variations in Insulin Response

Yalow and Berson showed that there were "great biological variations" in the "insulin secretory responses" of even healthy lean individuals. In response to ingesting *standard* quantities of glucose: individuals secrete varying amounts of insulin into the bloodstream; their insulin varies in its effectiveness at lowering blood sugar; and blood sugar remains elevated in the circulation for different amounts of time.

The extensive variations observed in glucose tolerance tests may reflect both genetic and environmental factors. To date it has been difficult to determine the extent to which genetic factors contribute to these biological variations. Further work in this area of biological variation is critical to understanding the differences between health and disease (diabetes) and the prevention of obesity and diabetes in our culture.

More progress has been made in understanding the environmental factors that exert dietary control. We will discuss these environmental factors in greater depth later in this book. For now, it is important to recognize that environmental factors like food affect the insulin mechanisms in the body and may exacerbate certain genetic tendencies.

Insulin Sensitivity

It is essential to recognize how effectively insulin blocks fat metabolism. Fat cells in adipose tissue are exquisitely sensitive to insulin. Even slight elevations of insulin will increase the accumulation of fat in these adipose cells. Furthermore, fat cells remain sensitive to insulin long after muscle cells have become resistant to insulin.

As insulin levels rise, the storage of fat in fat cells increases. However, the pancreas may compensate for insulin resistance by secreting even more insulin into the blood circulation. This further increases the insulin levels in the bloodstream and therefore further increases fat storage and obesity.

In other words, in this vicious cycle, fat storage stops only when insulin levels in the bloodstream return to normal levels. High calorie snacks, which usually contain an abundance of carbohydrates, prolong fat storage in the body by preventing insulin levels from returning to normal.

Insulin Resistance

Research by David Rabinowitz and Kenneth Zierler, endocrinologists at Johns Hopkins Medical School, corroborated Yalow and Berson's initial observations about insulin resistance. They showed that both type II diabetics and obese individuals had excesses of insulin in the blood and showed "greatly exaggerated" insulin responses to carbohydrate.

It took years before standardized tests for insulin resistance were developed. Stanford diabetologist, Gerald Reaven, and his associate, John Farquhar, published the first details of a test for insulin resistance. However, it took the work of Ralph Defronzo, who initially worked at the NIH and later was admitted to the faculty of Yale University School of Medicine, to refine the procedure. The details of this procedure were published in 1979, nearly 20 years after Yalow and Berson learned how to measure insulin in the blood stream. This led to a breakthrough in understanding the nature of Type II, or adult-onset, diabetes.

Developing a reliable measurement for insulin resistance was no small achievement. It required multiple tests for both blood insulin and blood sugar while insulin levels were held constant through the precise control of the glucose consumed by the subject. The results of this test, if conducted properly, would allow the investigator to determine how much insulin was necessary to deliver sugar from the blood stream into cells and tissues throughout the body of the subjects. If sugar-delivery processes required increased amounts of insulin compared to normal controls, the subject was deemed to be insulin resistant.

After 20 years, the medical establishment was finally able to recognize that insulin resistance was the fundamental defect in Type II diabetes.

Hormone Regulation of Fat Mobilization

Insulin blocks fat mobilization. Numerous other hormones promote fat mobilization. These include Epinephrine, Norepinephrine, Glucagon, Thyroid-stimulating hormone, Melanocyte-stimulating hormone, Vasopressin, and growth hormone. Nevertheless, the effects of insulin are so strong that even minor elevations in insulin can override these other hormones.

Neurotransmitters and Hormones Regulate Appetite

The Appetite Center

The appetite center is contained within the *Arcuate Nucleus* (ARC), which is centrally located in the brain stem on the ventral surface of the hypothalamus close to the median eminence. Within the ARC, two neuronal networks regulate appetite levels in different directions:

- Neuropeptide Y (NPY), ARP (Agouti-related protein) and Cannabinoids are *orexigenic*, meaning that they increase appetite.
- POMC (pro-opiomelanocortin), its peptide derivative (alpha MSH), and CART (Cocaine and amphetamine related transcripts) are *anorexigenic*, meaning they decrease appetite or provide satiety.[1]

There are also feedback loops that allow nerve fibers from the ARP network to communicate with the POMC network, thus decreasing the inhibitory fibers in the appetite center. This suggests that appetite stimulation predominates over appetite suppression, a characteristic that must have been important in the evolution of the human species by stimulating the search for food.

The appetite center also has neural projections directed to the ventro-medial hypothalamus and the lateral hypothalamus that connect with the paraventricular nucleus (PVN), the lateral hypothalamic area (LHA), the perifornical area (PFA), and the zona incerta (ZI).

Other projections are directed to the parasympathetic nervous system, mediated by acetylcholine, and to the sympathetic nervous system, mediated by adrenaline (epinephrine) and noradrenaline (norepinephrine). Activation of the parasympathetic nervous system is associated with food intake, digestion, and absorption. Activation of the sympathetic nervous system is associated with fight-and-flight responses by the musculoskeletal system. A central tenet of human physiology is that parasympathetic and sympathetic stimulation cannot be sustained at the same time.

The superchiasmatic nucleus, sensitized by daylight (blue light at 490 nm) as part of circadian rhythms, also releases a hormone, Orexin, that stimulates appetite in the Arcuate Nucleus.

The highly organized neural networks that interact in the appetite center and communicate with the hypothalamus and peripheral nerves (both parasympathetic and sympathetic nervous systems) indicate that appetite control is central to reproduction, growth, maturation, and survival of human beings. The hypothalamus is where the neural networks communicate with hormone-secreting cells that regulate the entire endocrine system throughout the body. Neuro-hormonal cascades in the brain regulate hormone secretion from the anterior and posterior pituitary glands, which in turn regulate the hormonal cascades of peripheral glands, including reproductive glands (ovaries and testes), stress glands (adrenal medulla and cortex), gastrointestinal glands (pancreatic islets and hormone secreting cells along the GI tract), metabolic glands (thyroid), and immune glands (thymus and bone marrow cells).

Neurotransmitters Regulate Appetite

The neurotransmitters and nerves that regulate the appetite center in the brain and project signals to the peripheral nervous system are shown in the table below as functions of two powerful regulatory cascades that either increase or decrease appetite:

Table 5-1

NEURAL NETWORK	HUNGER INCREASED (OREXIGENIC)	HUNGER DECREASED (ANOREXIGENIC)
Arcuate Nucleus(ARC)	NPY AgRP	POMC -> MSH CART
Hypothalamus	Projections into: - Paraventricular Nucleus (PVN) - Lateral Hypothalamic Area (LHA) - Perifornical Area (PFA) - Zona Incerta	Projections into: - Paraventricular Nucleus (PVN) - Lateral Hypothalamic Area (LHA) - Perifornical Area (PFA) - Zona Incerta
Peripheral nerves	Projections into Parasympathetic system: - Acetyl choline (Ach)	Projections into Sympathetic system: - Adrenaline (epinephrine) - Noradrenaline (norepinephrine)

Hormones Regulate Appetite

At the same time, hormonal signals from peripheral cells in the gastro-intestinal tract and fat cells regulate the neural networks in the appetite center to either increase (orexigenic) or decrease (anorexigenic) appetite levels. The principal hormones that affect appetite are shown in the table below:

Table 5-2

Hormone	Source of hormone	Effect on Appetite
Ghrelin	Stomach & intestinal tract	orexigenic
Peptide YY (PYY)	Intestinal tract	anorexigenic
Cholecystokinin (CCK)	Intestinal tract	anorexigenic
Leptin	Fat cells	anorexigenic

Ghrelin is secreted from endocrine cells in the stomach and intestinal tract in response to the absence of food. It is a powerful stimulant of appetite. It is the only appetite stimulant made outside the brain.

Peptide YY (PYY) is secreted from endocrine cells in the intestinal tract in response to food. As it circulates to the brain, it switches off the urge to eat.

Cholecystokinin (CCK) is secreted from endocrine cells lining the upper intestinal tract (the duodenum) in response to food particularly protein and fat. It therefore acts to decrease appetite.

Leptin is a hormone that is secreted by fat cells. Mice lacking Leptin (Leptin mutation) ate voraciously and grew enormously fat. Leptin injections made them stop eating and slim down. However, the effect of Leptin in humans is different. Most obese subjects have high levels of Leptin. Thus, the effect of Leptin in humans appears to be muted: obese humans eat despite high Leptin levels.

Summary

Insulin is the master switch that shifts fuel-utilization from fat-burning pathways to carbohydrate-burning pathways. Insulin itself blocks the metabolism of fat, which results in fat accumulation in fat pads. In this process, carbohydrate-rich diets lead to uncontrolled hunger and uncontrolled weight gain through high blood sugar, high blood insulin levels, and insulin resistance.

While hormones regulate energy shifts in the body, neurotransmitters in the brain and hormones from the digestive tract and fat depots regulate the appetite center (arcuate nucleus) in the brain stem.

The next several chapters focus on the metabolism of fat and carbohydrate in the body and further underscore the role of refined carbohydrates and sugars in causing excessive fat storage.

Chapter 6

Fat Distribution in the Body

The Importance of Body Fat

In today's vanity-conscious world, many people seek to lose weight simply to maintain an attractive figure. Weight loss has an aesthetic component in addition to its health benefits. Sometimes, this drives people to the extreme of seeking to eliminate fat entirely from their diets and their bodies. Before we can turn to the subject of weight loss and weight control, however, we need to understand that fat is necessary for human survival. Fat has several essential functions.

- Adipose tissue is necessary for the storage of fat-soluble vitamins
- Fat serves as long-term energy supplies. It contains 9 calories per gram of fat, more than twice as many calories as carbohydrate and protein, each of which contains only 4 calories per gram
- Adipose tissue improves the shape of human beings and confers on both women and men attractive figures that are important for maturation, reproduction, and evolution

In 1965, George Cahill and Albert Renold noted that "Survival of the [human] species must have depended many times both on the ability to store adequate yet not excessive amounts of energy in the form of fat, and on the ability of being able to mobilize these stores always at a sufficient rate to meet the body's needs." They added that at one time, the ideal amount of fat stored in the body "should be... sufficiently large to allow for periods of fasting to which a given species in a given environment is customarily exposed, yet sufficiently small to preserve maximum mobility." Optimally, a 150-pound man with 20% body fat would have stored enough fat to survive for two months of total starvation.

While that was true for eons, it is no longer true today. While we possess substantially the same metabolism that responded to periods of starvation in primitive times, we no longer experience a shortage of food in advanced societies. The result has been that the mechanisms that once preserved fat for the sake of survival are inappropriate in today's sedentary society and have led to enormous increases in overweight disorders and obesity.

Regulators of Fat Distribution in the Human Body

Lipoprotein Lipase (LPL)

A crucial enzyme in the fat distribution process is lipoprotein lipase, or LPL, which regulates the uptake of fatty acids throughout the body. When lipoprotein-rich particles pass through the circulation, the LPL enzyme will bind with triglycerides in these particles and breakdown the triglycerides into their component parts: fatty acids and glycerol phosphate. This increases the free fatty acids that can be taken up into the cell to be stored as triglycerides or oxidized for energy production.

Not surprisingly, insulin regulates LPL activity, though it does so differently depending on the kind of cell involved. Insulin increases LPL activity and fat storage in fat cells, while it decreases LPL activity in muscle tissue and stimulates the muscles to burn glucose. Decreases in insulin reduce LPL activity and uptake of fatty acids into fat cells. At the same time LPL activity and uptake of fatty acids are stimulated in muscle cells. This is part of the Randle cycle that we discussed in chapter 4.

Differential Distribution of Fat in Men and Women

The distribution of LPL in body tissues determines why men and women show fat-distribution patterns that are different. Women have greater LPL activity in their adipose tissue than men do, and this may account for why women have a greater predisposition to weight gains than men do. Women have more LPL activity in the hips and buttocks than in the abdominal region, although after menopause the LPL activity in the abdominal region catches up with men. On the other hand, men have more LPL activity in the abdominal region, which may explain why men put on more belly fat.

Regulators of LPL Distribution

Knowing the regulators of LPL distribution helps us understand the measures that are necessary to lose weight and achieve weight control. Obese people have heightened LPL activity in their fat cells, a condition that may be due to the stimulating effects of excess insulin levels in the bloodstream. Exercise increases LPL activity in muscle tissue, enhancing the uptake and oxidation of fatty acids during muscular activity. Under sedentary conditions, however, the reverse occurs and LPL activity increases in fat tissue.

Under conditions of growth, maturation, and reproduction, LPL activity can be mediated by reproductive hormones like estrogen, progesterone, and testosterone. In women, progesterone increases LPL activity in the hips and buttocks. Estrogen decreases LPL activity, which may explain why women put on weight after menopause, when estrogen levels decrease. In men, testosterone initially suppresses LPL activity in the abdomen, which may explain why men put on weight around the midsection as they age.

Diets rich in carbohydrates increase the LPL activity in fat tissue. By contrast, fat-rich diets show no changes in LPL activity. It is likely that insulin serves as the predominant regulator of LPL activity in fat tissue and that sex hormones regulate the distribution of fat throughout the body in gender-specific patterns.

The uptake of free fatty acids in the liver is regulated by a different enzyme, Hepatic Lipase. Although it functions in a similar manner to process and absorb fatty acids from dietary triglycerides in the portal system, it shows little or no regulation by sex hormones.

Proteins Regulate Adipogenesis

Intracellular and extracellular proteins appear to regulate the size of adipose tissue by a process known as adipogenesis. For example, the Sirtuin family of seven cellular proteins has recently been shown to be important in the control of aging and metabolism[1]. Sirt2 is the most abundant of the Sirtuins in fat cells. It is expressed in quantities five to ten times higher than the other Sirtuin proteins. When persons gain weight, cells in connective tissue known as pre-adipocytes differentiate and fill with fat and form adipocytes (fat cells), which are able to store fat as a potential source of energy when food is not available. However, too much fat storage leads to obesity and to many obesity-related diseases, including type II diabetes.

Using genetically altered cells from mice, Joslin Diabetes Center researchers were able to manipulate Sirt2 levels in adipocytes. They found that increasing Sirt2 levels in the cell would block the cell's ability to undergo differentiation and store fat, while reducing Sirt2 would promote adipogenesis or fat production.

Thus, when Sirt2 levels in pre-adipocytes are low, more fat cells develop, while when Sirt2 levels are high, this process is blocked. "So, to reduce the amount of fat in the body and help people stay thin, we need to find an activator of Sirt2," said Dr. C. Ronald Kahn, who is head of the Joslin Section on Obesity and Hormone Action at Harvard Medical School.

Extracellular proteins or hormones may also protect the body from excessive formation of adipose tissue and the effects of type II diabetes. Adiponectin, produced in fat cells, may improve insulin sensitivity and reduce cardiovascular risk, according to Osama Hamdy, Medical Director of the Obesity Clinical Program at the Joslin Diabetes Center in Boston.[2]

Type II Diabetes and Adipogenesis

Other studies in the Joslin Diabetes Center indicate that fat-cell adipose tissues may be considered an endocrine organ. Fat-cell adipocytes secrete prohormones and cytokines, including adiponectin, leptin, TNF-alpha, IL-6, resistin, and plasminogen activator inhibitor. High levels of proinflammatory cytokines, including TNF-alpha, are related to insulin resistance, atherosclerosis, and coronary artery disease. Most cytokines are produced not only by the fat cells but also by the macrophages in the fat tissue. Macrophages are attracted to areas of fat cell necrosis that occur in older and obese patients, according to Hamdy.

Removal of subcutaneous fat in humans undergoing liposuction procedures did not change blood pressure, lipid abnormalities, glucose tolerance, C-reactive protein, TNF-alpha, or adiponectin. However, removal of visceral fat in mice did improve glucose tolerance. These findings have given rise to the hypothesis that visceral fat and subcutaneous fat have different regulatory features related to the onset of Type II diabetes. However, this hypothesis must be validated by additional studies.

Dr. Hamdy explains that the standard model of diabetes care has been focused on management of Hemoglobin A1c, the glycation derivative of the hemoglobin protein in the blood circulation. However, Dr. Hamdy recommends that the focus of diabetic care be concentrated on reduction of body weight. Dr. Hamdy recommends that type II diabetics reduce their carbohydrate intake to 40% of calories and maintain a protein intake of 30% calories, which leaves fat intake at 30% of calories.

Given the conversion rates of grams to calories for carbohydrate (4 calories per gram), protein (4 calories per gram), and fat (9 calories per gram), the Hamby diet, based on 2000 total calories, would look like this:

Table 6-1

Food type	% Calories	Total Calories	Grams
Carbohydrate	40%	800	200 g
Protein	30%	600	150 g
Fat	30%	600	66 g

This is a high-protein, moderately low-carbohydrate and low-fat diet which, according to Dr. Hamdy, should be used along with strength training and cognitive behavior training. Substantial benefits were observed with type II diabetic patients over a 3-month period, as follows:

- People in the program lost an average of 24.6 pounds
- Waist circumference declined by 3.7 inches
- Average hemoglobin A1c levels declined to less than 7.0 (82% of subjects achieved normal hemoglobin A1c levels)
- Lipid profiles and blood pressure improved
- Significant declines were observed in cytokines, C-Reactive Protein, and TNF-alpha, along with a significant increase in adiponectin
- Diabetes medication was reduced by 50 to 60%
- Patients saved about $560 in diabetes medications per year

The conclusion of this study, which focused on reduction of body weight, showed the following improvements in patient care:

- Diabetes medication was reduced
- Cost was lowered
- A1c goals were achieved
- Coronary artery disease risk was significantly reduced
- Quality of life was improved.

Drugs and Adipogenesis

Selective serotonin receptor inhibitors (SSRI), which are used to treat depression disorders, are notorious for increasing body weight. The following SSRIs are the greatest offenders, some adding more than 100 pounds to body weight: Celexa, Cymbalta, Effexor, Lexapro, Paxil, Prozac, Risperdal, Sarafem, Wellbutrin, Zoloft, and Zyprexa.

Some anti-diabetic medications may add more than 70 pounds, including Thiazolidinedione (TZD), which increases the body's sensitivity to insulin, and Sulfonylureas, which causes the pancreas to release more insulin.

White Versus Brown Fat

There are two types of fat cells with different functions: the well-known fat cells, which store energy and contribute to obesity, and the lesser-known brown fat cells, which burn calories to generate body heat. Although humans are born with a good supply of brown fat cells, these are usually diminished after infancy. The loss of brown fat cells may be related to the loss of a selective advantage for humans to enter into hibernation under low-temperature conditions once the species learned how to avoid extreme temperatures through housing and heating technologies that provided sustained temperature controls.

Three recent studies indicate that humans contain vestiges of the brown fat cells that are important in animals, like bears, whales and penguins for hibernation. Brown fat acts like a furnace, consuming calories and generating heat. Brown fat cells have a darker color than white fat cells because they contain greater numbers of mitochondria that provide energy to the cell. Mitochondria are rich in iron, giving the tissue its reddish-brown color.

The breakthrough in demonstrating that humans have functioning brown fat cells was made possible by PET-CT scans. This radiological procedure can visualize brown fat depots because these cells rapidly burn glucose to produce heat. This increase in metabolic activity lights up the PET scans and identifies the locations of brown fat reserves. Furthermore, exposure to cold environments, such as 61 degrees Fahrenheit for 2 hours, further activates brown fat cells, according to studies conducted in Sweden and the Netherlands.

In humans, the vestige of brown fat tissue appears in the upper back, along the sides of the neck, along the spine, and along the collarbone to the shoulder. Human infants show increased brown fat depots as sheets covering their backs. Thinner people have more brown fat than heavier people, younger people more than older people, and women more than men. People with lower glucose levels also show more brown fat depots, suggesting they have higher metabolic rates than those with sluggish metabolism.

Bruce Spiegelman at the Dana Farber Cancer Institute discovered that brown fat cells can be made from the same precursor tissues that normally produce muscle cells. "Brown fat can increase energy production and protect against obesity," Spiegelman writes. "The epidemic of obesity, closely associated with increases in diabetes, hypertension, hyperlipidemia, cancer and other disorders, has propelled a major interest in adipose cells and tissues." The next step, he says, "is to find specific drugs and techniques that could help the body make more brown fat cells or else genetically engineer white fat cells to turn brown."

Lipoprotein Particles Transport Fat and Cholesterol in the Blood Stream

Oil and water do not mix. The same is true of fatty acids and triglycerides (oily lipids) in the bloodstream (water). The body has had to evolve complex enzymatic systems to move fatty acids and triglycerides through the bloodstream not as fat, but as lipoprotein particles. Protein and cholesterol act as surfactants (surface agents) that allow for lipoprotein particles to remain soluble in the blood circulation. For this reason, the scientific investigation of lipid intake, transfer, storage, and utilization has been more difficult than the study of carbohydrates and sugars, which are freely soluble in body fluids, including blood.

It may seem ironic that a medical physicist who employed ultracentrifuges to purify uranium in World War II as part of the Manhattan Project for the ultimate construction of the atomic bomb would become the central figure who initiated research on lipoprotein particles after the war. However, in the late 1940s, while on the faculty of the University of California at Berkeley, John Gofman applied his knowledge of centrifuges to the purification of lipoprotein particles that circulate through the bloodstream. This line of research would ultimately launch the modern era of cholesterol research by enriching our understanding of the role of lipoprotein particles in atherosclerosis, heart disease, and obesity.

In 1950, Gofman published his groundbreaking work, "The Role of Lipids and Lipoproteins in Atherosclerosis." Cholesterol, Gofman noted, is only one of several fatlike substances that circulate in blood. Collectively, blood lipids combine with protein to form the lipoprotein particles that transport triglycerides to target tissues for storage or metabolism.

Gofman's research called into question the wisdom of gauging heart disease merely by the amount of cholesterol in the bloodstream. Very Low Density Lipoproteins (VLDL) and Low Density Lipoproteins (LDL), Gofman concluded, are equally important variables. Gofman proposed an "atherogenic" index that added measures of the two particles together and produced a better predictor of atherosclerosis and heart disease.

Gofman's studies clearly demonstrated that while the amount of LDL in the blood can be elevated by the consumption of saturated fats, the amount of VLDL that contains most of the triglycerides in the blood is elevated by carbohydrate. These findings led to the conclusion that VLDL can be lowered *only* when carbohydrate consumption is reduced.

Ultimately, researchers came to identify the different classes of lipoprotein particles according to their density. From low density to high, these lipoproteins are VLDL (very low-density lipoproteins), LDL (low-density lipoproteins), SDL (small, dense lipoproteins), and HDL (high-density lipoproteins). Let us begin by examining how these four lipoprotein particles function in transporting triglycerides (fat) and cholesterol throughout the body.

VLDL: Very Low Density Lipoproteins

Most of the dietary triglycerides are carried on lipoprotein particles. Triglycerides are initially secreted from hepatocytes in the liver as VLDL particles. They are called very low density because they are packed with low-density triglycerides. As with all lipoprotein particles, the lipid content is surrounded by phospholipids, cholesterol, and a protein called apo B. The protein/lipid coat allows the lipid particles to remain soluble in the bloodstream and the interstitial space around tissue cells. The surface coating of phospholipids, cholesterol, and apo B carries the triglycerides to tissues throughout the body, where it drops them off in a process known as "delipidation."

As VLDL particles release their triglycerides, the particles decrease in size, their density increases and they become LDL particles. These LDL particles continue to release triglycerides, and they become small, low–density LDL particles (SDL). VLDL is therefore commonly referred to as a "precursor" of LDL and LDL the precursor for SDL.

Carbohydrate-Induced Lipemia

Lipemia is the condition of abnormally high levels of triglycerides (fat) in the bloodstream. After the blood cells are sedimented in this condition, the serum appears to the naked eye to contain high concentrations of VLDL, the largest fat (lipoprotein) particles. Hence the name "lipemia," or high lipid concentrations in the blood or serum. Dietary carbohydrate appears to regulate the amount of VLDL in the serum. Increasing carbohydrate in the diet increases VLDL levels, which are correlated with increased risk of heart disease. On the other hand, decreasing carbohydrate in the diet decreases LDL levels and decreases VLDL levels even more.

As shown by Pete Ehrens and Margaret Albrink at the Rockefeller University in the 1960s, elevated triglyceride levels were far more likely to be present than high cholesterol levels in patients with coronary-heart disease. In one study, 82% of coronary patients had high triglyceride levels. By comparison, only 5% of healthy young men and 38% of healthy middle-aged men showed high levels of triglycerides.

By 1970, independent researchers around the world had confirmed that high triglycerides were associated far more strongly than cholesterol with heart disease. One study, conducted by Lars Carlson, Peter Kuo, and Joseph Goldstein, reported that lipemia induced by carbohydrate consumption accounted for 90% of the incidence of high cholesterol. Further, when patients were put on a sugar-free diet containing only 500 to 600 calories of starch a day, their triglyceride and cholesterol levels were significantly reduced.

Beginning in 1967 Donald Frederickson, Robert Levy, and Robert Lees devised an inexpensive technique for measuring the triglycerides and cholesterol in lipoprotein particles fractionated by using an analytical centrifuge. They identified five lipoprotein disorders in humans, designating them with Roman numerals. Out of these five disorders, by far the most common was Type IV, a carbohydrate-induced lipemia that was signaled by elevated VLDL triglycerides. The "sizeable fraction" of coronary patients with Type IV disorders could be treated only with low-carbohydrate diets.

LDL: Low Density Lipoproteins (Bad Cholesterol)

The amount of LDL does not accurately reflect the amount of cholesterol in the blood, even though LDL carries 70% of the total cholesterol. High levels of LDL are more prevalent in patients with atherosclerosis than in healthy subjects, in men more than in women, and in older individuals more than in younger, and it is regularly found in diabetics.

In the 1980s Krauss extended the density gradient studies of Gofman and found that LDL particles may be subfractionated into seven discrete subclasses that fall into two distinct patterns or traits, called pattern A and pattern B. Pattern A is characterized by large, fluffy LDL and is accompanied by low triglycerides and high HDL. Pattern A poses a low risk for heart disease. By contrast, Pattern B is characterized by small, dense LDL (SDL), which correlates with atherosclerotic heart disease. This pattern is invariably accompanied by high triglyceride and low HDL levels. In fact, heart disease patients were three times more likely to have pattern B than A. Pattern B is called the atherogenic profile, which is also found in diabetics.

SDL: Small, Dense Lipoprotein Particles (Very Bad Cholesterol)

Further research is needed to understand why normal individuals readily metabolize small, dense LDL particles while individuals with heart disease have difficulty metabolizing these particles. The relative dearth of cholesterol in these particles may cause structural changes that promote plaque formation in arterial walls. The longevity of SDL particles in the blood stream may lead to glycation and oxidation products that are internalized by the macrophages that contribute to plague formation. And small, dense LDL may oxidize more readily than large, low-density particles that contain more cholesterol and triglycerides.

HDL: High Density Lipoproteins (Good Cholesterol)

The hypothesis that HDL particles protect against heart disease had first been proposed in 1951 by David Barr and Howard Eder of New York Hospital-Cornell Medical Center. In John Gofman's last paper, he confirmed the existence of cholesterol-containing HDL particles and showed that when HDL was low, triglycerides tended to be high and vice versa. This suggested that the two parameters were linked.

Later studies questioned whether *total* cholesterol was a risk factor at all for heart disease. LDL cholesterol was a "marginal" risk factor. Rather, they singled out triglycerides as the most important risk factor. For men and women 50 years or older, HDL was the only reliable predictor of heart disease risk in men and women.

In 1977, Tavia Gordon and her associates concluded that anything that raised HDL appears to lower triglycerides and vice versa. "This suggests that physical activity, weight loss and a low carbohydrate intake may be beneficial," Gordon and her collaborators wrote. It is ironic that they published their conclusions only three days after George McGovern's Senate Select Committee on Nutrition and Human Needs concluded that the best diet to prevent heart disease was one low in fat and high in carbohydrates.

Summary

This chapter explains how the body has solved the difficulty of mixing oil and water in transporting fat through the aqueous medium of the blood circulation. The body has evolved cofactors, including proteins, phospholipids and cholesterol that serve to encapsulate fat particles during their transport through the blood. The release of triglycerides from these lipoprotein particles depends on specific enzymes, including lipoprotein lipase and hepatic lipase, in target cells.

The distributions of these lipid-absorbing enzymes in target cellular membranes is determined genetically and accounts for the differential distribution of fat in men and women. The role of reproductive hormones in modulating the amounts of fat-absorbing enzymes, accounts for many of the changes in fat distribution seen as a function of age and reproductive health in both genders.

Now that we understand how fat is ingested, transferred, stored, and metabolized in both men and women, we need to understand further why refined carbohydrates and sugar are so toxic.

Chapter 7

Sugar: Pure, Sweet, and Deadly

Per-Capita Rise in Sugar Consumption

In chapter 2 we discussed Cleave's and Campbell's hypothesis that westernized diets containing sugar, white flour, and white rice are primarily responsible for the appearance of the "diseases of civilization," including obesity, diabetes, coronary heart disease, and gallbladder disease, and possibly cancer as well. John Yudkin concluded that high-sugar diets led to high cholesterol, triglyceride, and insulin levels. Yudkin added that sugar and starches brought little of nutritional value to the diet except for fuel calories that could be burned for energy. He believed that sugar was the worst offender, so he recommended that sugar be the first substance removed from the diet of overweight individuals.

In Chapter 2, we saw that the greatest single change in the American diet over the past two centuries has been the dramatic increase in the average yearly consumption of sugar in the United States, as the table below shows.

Table 7-1

Period	Sugar consumption per capita
1830	15 lbs
1920	100 lbs
1960	110 lbs
1975	124 lbs
2000	150 lbs[1]

Chemistry of Complex Carbohydrates and Sugars

It is now important to review the chemistry of simple sugars and complex carbohydrates. Simple carbohydrates (refined sugars), as in sucrose produced from sugar cane, are molecules of one or two sugars chemically bound together. Complex carbohydrates, as in the starches contained in flour, pasta, noodles, bread, potatoes and pizza, may be tens of thousands of sugars long.

The carbohydrates in starch are broken down by digestion, first into maltose and then into glucose, which is absorbed from the small intestine into the bloodstream. Complex carbohydrates take considerably longer to be broken down and digested in the intestinal track than a simple sugar like sucrose (cane sugar), which is composed of glucose and fructose molecules linked together in a short disaccharide chain, and lactose, which is composed of glucose and galactose in a short disaccharide chain.

Glycemic Index

In the 1970s David Jenkins and Thomas Wolever, both at Oxford University, refined the study of glycemic index, which is a measure of how fully carbohydrates are digested and absorbed into the circulation and converted into blood sugar 2 hours after ingestion. They tested 62 foods and recorded the blood sugar response two hours after consumption of 100 grams. A standard solution of glucose was used as a benchmark and assigned a numerical a value of 100[1].

The glycemic index measures how readily carbohydrates are broken down in the digestion process and converted into blood sugar. The higher the index, the more the response resembles that from pure glucose.

Table 7-2 below lists the glycemic indices of several common, high-carbohydrate foods.

Table 7-2: Glycemic Index

Food	Glycemic index
Glucose	100
White bread	70
Saltines	74
Plain bagel	72
White rice	72
Corn flakes	83
Oatmeal	48
Sweet corn	56
French fries	75
Whole milk	30
Plain yogurt	14
Apples	38
Bananas	56
Vanilla ice cream	60

[1]Includes high fructose corn syrup (HFCS)

One point that needs to be emphasized is that the higher the carbohydrate content of a food, the greater the consequences for rise in blood sugar and insulin. Food processing practices such as the polishing of rice, the mashing of potatoes, the refining of wheat, and the use of simple sugars in soft drinks and fruit juices effectively increase the speed of digestion of carbohydrates as well as the glycemic index of the food.

High Fructose Corn Syrup (HFCS)

In 1978 high fructose corn syrup (HFCS) was introduced into the market. Because this type of sugar could be refined from corn rather than sugar cane or beets, the production costs were dramatically decreased. HFCS-55, with 55% fructose and 45% glucose, was created to mimic the taste of sucrose in soft drinks. However, HFCS-55, with the combination of two sugar molecules (glucose and fructose), will be absorbed more quickly than sucrose (glucose linked to fructose as a dissacharide), which requires digestion before the two sugars may be absorbed into the body. By 1985, half of the sugars consumed each year in the U.S. came from corn sweeteners.

Fructose, or "fruit sugar," is often mistakenly considered healthier than sucrose. Because of its low glycemic index of 22, fructose has also been mistakenly considered to be "safe" sugar. For example, an apple contains roughly 6% fructose, 4% sucrose, and 1% glucose. For this reason, HFCS is the primary sweetener used in sports drinks, fruit juices, and low-fat yogurt, foods that many children consume, often with their parents' consent. Unfortunately, scientific studies have indicated that fructose is far from safe. In fact, in numerous ways, it has been shown to be more toxic than glucose.

Within the liver, fructose is converted into glycerol phosphate more efficiently than glucose, a process that promotes the formation of triglycerides (fats). These triglycerides are then shipped out, in the form of lipoprotein particles, to fat depots in the body. Fructose is therefore considered the most lipogenic sugar.

Fructose also raises blood pressure disproportionately more than glucose. This is not new. It has been known since the 1960s.

Moreover, fructose is considered 10 times more harmful than glucose because it induces the non-specific cross-linking of proteins that lead to cellular precipitates related to dangerous advanced glycation end products (AGEs). Furthermore, those AGEs that have been formed with fructose are more resistant to cellular disposal processes than those formed with glucose. Fructose also seems to contribute to the development of atherosclerosis by accelerating the oxidation of LDL. The subjects of protein glycation and advanced glycation end products appears in the next chapter.

The Differences among Sucrose, Glucose, and Fructose

Table sugar, refined from sugar cane, is composed of sucrose, a disaccharide containing a single glucose molecule linked to a single fructose molecule. Following the digestion of sucrose in the intestinal tract, glucose moves into the bloodstream and raises blood sugar, which is then utilized by all the peripheral organs and tissues in the body. By contrast, fructose can be metabolized only by the liver. Fructose therefore has little effect on carbohydrate metabolism outside the liver. Consequently, only the glucose portion of sucrose is reflected in the glycemic index. However, these findings do not make fructose a "better" sugar than glucose.

The Harmful Effects of Sugar and HFCS

The food industry adds enormous quantities of sugar to liquid beverages. In almost every case, the amount of sugar added far exceeds the sugar contained in the apple, orange, or pear that might otherwise be the snack of choice. Even worse, sugar is addictive; many consumers will reach for two, three, or more of these drinks a day. Profit margins are so high that fast-food restaurants promote super-sized soft drinks. At 64 ounces, these drinks add 160 grams and 640 calories to the diet with virtually negligible cost to the restaurant. A single drink could account for one quarter to one third of the daily caloric requirements for growing children.

Consider three staples of the soft drink industry in Table 7-3.

This massive dose of sucrose is broken down rapidly into glucose and fructose by the intestine, and both sugars are rapidly absorbed into the blood. This amount of sugar provides a gross overload to the insulin system in the body, leading to hyperglycemia, hyperinsulinemia, and insulin resistance, three processes that ultimately lead to type II diabetes.

When HFCS-55 is used as an inexpensive replacement for sucrose, neither the glucose nor the fructose requires digestive steps; they therefore

Table 7-3

Product	Size	Total Sugar (Sucrose or HFCS)	Glucose	Fructose	Calories
Fruit Juice	8 oz	20 g	10 g	10 g	80
Soft drink	12 oz	30 g	15 g	15 g	120
Soft drink	64 oz	160 g	80 g	80 g	640

are absorbed even more rapidly, providing an even greater toxic jolt to the insulin system in the body.

Furthermore the more rapidly the blood sugar rises, the more rapidly the subsequent fall of sugar occurs, leading to symptoms of hypoglycemia, such as intense hunger, nausea, rapid heart rate, dizziness, and sweating. In our fast food culture, this encourages the consumption of yet another soft drink, which further compounds the problem.

There is no question that adding large amounts of refined sugars to soft drinks and fruit juice products continues to cause enormous harm to individuals. Not only are toxic effects such as wild swings in blood sugar and insulin levels experienced within hours of ingestion, but the continued over-consumption of refined sugar leads to toxic metabolic reactions in the body, including obesity, type II diabetes, Metabolic Syndrome, and ultimately the atherosclerosis that leads to cardiovascular disease and eventual heart attacks, strokes, peripheral vascular diseases, and premature mortality.

But the story gets worse. Fructose and glucose work synergistically in deleterious ways to create greater harm. Fructose interferes with the body's natural processes for metabolizing glucose and converting glucose into glycogen. Over time, high fructose diets affect insulin and blood sugar levels, encouraging insulin resistance, increasing the production of triglycerides, and indirectly promoting high blood pressure.

Together, the synergistic and deleterious effects of glucose and fructose may target sucrose and HFCS as Public Enemies Number 1 and Number 2 in the promotion of the Metabolic Syndrome, which is associated with the risk factors of obesity, glucose intolerance, hyperinsulinemia, insulin resistance, high triglycerides, low HDL levels, and elevated small, dense LDL particles.

Sugar Addiction

Not only is sugar, containing glucose and fructose, harmful to the body, it can also lead to an addictive disorder. Professor Bart Hoebel and his colleagues at the Neuroscience Institute at Princeton University have shown discrete symptoms of addiction when rats are fed high levels of sucrose in their water.

First, the rats became dependent on high doses of sugar. When the rats were denied sugar for prolonged periods after learning to binge on sugar, they showed signs of addiction, because they worked harder to get the sugar when it was reintroduced to them. They also consumed higher levels of sugar than ever before, suggesting craving and relapse behavior.

Binging on sugar provoked a surge of dopamine release in a region of the hungry rat's brain known as the *nucleus accumbens*, a finding that is reminiscent of drug addiction disorders. After a month, the structure of the brains of these experimental subjects had adapted to increased dopamine levels, showing fewer dopamine receptors than they used to have and more opioid receptors.

Signs of sugar withdrawal were shown among the rats after researchers took away their sugar supply. As their brain levels of dopamine dropped, the rats showed signs of anxiety and withdrawal. Their teeth chattered, and they were unwilling to navigate or explore simple maze structures in comparison to control littermates that were not exposed to sugar.

Rats eating large amounts of sugar when hungry underwent neuro-chemical changes in the brain that appeared to mimic those produced by substances of abuse, including cocaine, morphine, and nicotine. For example, the rats drank more alcohol than normal after their sugar supply was cut off, and they showed hyperactive behavior after receiving a minimal dose of amphetamines that had no effect on normal rats.

The long-term effects of sugar addiction, leading to paths of destructive behavior, are typical for substance-abuse disorders. This work provides compelling links between the development of abnormal desires for natural substances like sugar and traditionally defined substance-abuse disorders, such as drug addiction.

Summary

Refined sugars—glucose, fructose, sucrose, and high fructose corn syrup—in excessive concentrations over prolonged periods of time, show deadly effects on human health. In this chapter we explain the chemical differences between refined sugar and starch, how quickly they are digested and absorbed into the body and the consequences of each type of sugar on parameters of body health.

We also call attention to recent studies that have demonstrated that high levels of sugar in laboratory animals, over prolonged periods of time, lead to addictive disorders that can only be relieved by binging on high-sugar drinks at more frequent intervals throughout the day. Further, sugar addictions lead to the rapid development of carbohydrate toxicity and other addictions as well, including alcohol and drug addictions.

In the next chapter we will examine the consequences of the Metabolic Syndrome and see the degree to which excessive carbohydrate metabolism leads to pathological states that may be responsible, in part, for the risk factors associated with this metabolic disorder, which gives rise to a number of chronic degenerative diseases that are associated with accelerated aging and early death.

Part 3

The Metabolic Syndrome, Aging, and the Paradoxes of Nutritional Disease and Weight Control

"In spite of our efforts, we are still very far from the absolute truth and it is probable, especially in the biological sciences, that it will never be given us to see it in its nakedness. But this need not discourage us, for we are constantly nearing it. And moreover, with the help of our experiments, we grasp relations between phenomena which, though partial and relative, allow us more and more to extend our power over nature."

– Claude Bernard

Chapter 8

Metabolic Syndrome, Obesity,
and Accelerated Aging

Syndrome X (Metabolic Syndrome)

Gerald Reaven gave the prestigious Banting Lecture at the 1988 American Diabetes Association Meeting. During this lecture, he identified a collection of related disorders that he named "Syndrome X." These disorders shared connections to Type II diabetes, obesity, and heart disease. They included hyperglycemia (high blood sugar), hyperinsulinemia (high blood insulin levels), insulin resistance, high triglycerides, low HDL cholesterol, and high blood pressure. What made Reaven's research so remarkable was that it demonstrated that none of these disorders existed as isolated entities. All were interconnected through metabolism in ways medicine had never imagined.

Fourteen years later, in 2002, the National Cholesterol Education Program recognized Syndrome X and gave it "official" status by renaming it the "Metabolic Syndrome." Defining the Syndrome was a breakthrough in understanding the causes of chronic degenerative disease and accelerated aging. The Metabolic Syndrome is now understood to be associated with a battery of major chronic degenerative diseases, all of which lead to accelerated aging and early death. These include overweight disorders and obesity; high blood pressure; high cholesterol and triglycerides; high blood sugar and type II diabetes; cardiovascular disease, including heart attack and stroke; a variety of cancers, including breast, prostate, endometrial, and colon; osteoarthritis; and gallbladder disease.

Clinical Risk Factors

While the underlying causes of the syndrome are in dispute, the Mayo Clinic has identified the clinical signs or risk factors that point to the Metabolic Syndrome. The first is age. Fewer than 10% of people in their 20s suffer from Metabolic Syndrome, but 40% of people in their 60s do. A second is race. While the syndrome affects people of all races, it seems to pose a greater risk for Hispanics and Asians. The third is obesity. Overweight individuals with a body mass index greater than 25 are increasingly at risk of Metabolic Syndrome. People with a family history of type II diabetes or a history of diabetes during pregnancy have increased chances of developing Metabolic Syndrome. Other risk factors include high blood pressure and cardiovascular disease, both of which are associated with an increased risk. A final factor is smoking, which increases insulin resistance and exacerbates the consequences of the Metabolic Syndrome.

Metabolic Syndrome puts people especially at risk of life-threatening coronary heart disease, stroke, and peripheral vascular disease. Among the consequences of Metabolic Syndrome are hyperglycemia, hyperinsulinemia, insulin resistance, and blood lipid disorders, including high triglycerides, low HDL cholesterol, and high LDL cholesterol. All of these risk factors contribute to inflammation and plaque buildup in artery walls, which contribute to atherosclerotic (plaque) disease.

Diagnosis

While there are no precise criteria for diagnosing the metabolic syndrome at the present time, the American Heart Association and the National Heart, Lung, and Blood Institute recommend that the metabolic syndrome be identified as the presence of three or more of the following components:

- Elevated waist size: for men, a circumference equal to 40 inches or greater; for women, 35 inches or greater
- Elevated triglycerides (150 mg/dL or greater)
- Reduced HDL ("good") cholesterol: for men, lower than 40 mg/Dl; For women, lower than 50 mg/dL
- Elevated blood pressure equal to or greater than 130/85 mm Hg
- Elevated fasting glucose equal to or greater than 100 mg/dL

Treatment

Currently, the medical profession treats the risk factors associated with Metabolic Syndrome with pharmaceutical agents designed to treat individual symptoms. These may include weight-loss medications, blood pressure medications, cholesterol medications, insulin-resistance medications, anti-thrombotic medications, blood thinning agents, anti-depressant medications, sleep medications, and anti-anxiety medications. Unfortunately, many of these substances have interacting and cumulative side effects that can actually exacerbate the aging process associated with Metabolic Syndrome.

Doctors also recommend aggressive lifestyle changes, including increased physical activity, losing weight, and quitting smoking, all of which should help reduce blood pressure and improve cholesterol and blood sugar levels, three key measures of metabolic distress. They may also advocate specific dietary changes to address different aspects of the syndrome. Among these are reducing saturated fat intake to lower insulin resistance, reducing sodium intake to lower blood pressure, and reducing high-glycemic carbohydrates to lower triglyceride levels.

Continuum of Metabolic Disorders

As part of the Metabolic Syndrome, cardiovascular degeneration appears to be caused by disturbances in carbohydrate and fat metabolism that lead to a battery of metabolic abnormalities, including high blood sugar, high insulin, insulin resistance, high triglycerides, low HDL, and elevated small, dense LDL particles.

These pathological conditions, all of which lead to atherosclerosis, appear to be operating in all of us. While those with Type II diabetes are further along the curve toward accelerated cardiovascular disease, everyone is moving along the same curve, some more rapidly than others. Seen in its full spectrum, the metabolic continuum defines a pathway from normal individuals to individuals suffering from Metabolic Syndrome to individuals suffering from Type II diabetes and/or cardiovascular disease.

The National Institutes of Health define the risk factors and diseases associated with the Metabolic Syndrome as follows:

- Overweight disorders and obesity
- High blood pressure
- High cholesterol and triglycerides levels
- Pre-diabetes with High blood sugar
- Type 2 diabetes
- Cardiovascular disease (heart attack and stroke)

- Certain cancers (breast, prostate, endometrial, colon)
- Osteoarthritis
- Gallbladder disease

In addition many patients with these chronic degenerative diseases also suffer from hyperthrombotic states, increased non-specific body inflammation, chronic stress, depression, anxiety and sleep disorders including sleep apnea.

It is important to note that overweight disorders and obesity often presage many of the other risk factors and diseases associated with the Metabolic Syndrome. Consequently, individuals who are overweight should be checked by their doctors for the presence of other metabolic disorders and diseases as well.

There is increasing evidence that excessive carbohydrate consumption is a major cause of the Metabolic Syndrome. Despite the dedication of cardiologists over the past 60 years to the high fat/cholesterol hypothesis of Ancel Keys, the evidence increasingly points to high carbohydrate intake, not fat, as the culprit. Epidemiological studies have shown successful weight loss through dietary changes and examined the nutritional causes of the "diseases of civilization," including obesity. Physiological studies have applied modern cellular and molecular biology techniques to the study of fuel distribution, storage, and energy utilization within the body. These support the conclusion that high carbohydrate consumption, not high fat consumption, is a major contributor in the development of the Metabolic Syndrome.

The rate of "acceleration" of Metabolic Syndrome is known to be determined by multi-factorial processes related to genetic endowments, inherited from parents through long lineages of ancestor populations. In the case of existing disease, the rate of acceleration is also determined by good medical treatment. For example, numerous studies have shown that good management of blood glucose levels through the careful administration of insulin prolongs the life of diabetic patients.

What is less well recognized, however, is that the rate of acceleration of Metabolic Syndrome is also determined by nutritional factors in the diet. Indeed, regulating metabolic processes nutritionally can help avoid the secondary and tertiary consequences of carbohydrate as well as fat metabolism, both of which accelerate the aging process that is associated with the Metabolic Syndrome.

The Metabolic Syndrome, Insulin, and Atherosclerosis

Evidence is now mounting that insulin plays a pivotal role, not only in the development of obesity, but also in the development of atherosclerosis. Based on the molecular dynamics of food intake and carbohydrate pathways for fuel distribution, it now appears likely that excessive secretion of insulin, induced by the consumption of refined carbohydrates and sugars, might be responsible for the development of atherosclerosis and cardiovascular disease in normal individuals.

Let us re-examine the cholesterol experiments conducted in rabbits in 1949.

- Rabbits that were fed high-cholesterol diets developed atherosclerotic plaques throughout their arteries. Ironically, this study was used initially to support the high-cholesterol, high-fat hypothesis promoted by Ancel Keys. However, what was lost in the interpretation of these experiments was the fact that 70% of the calories delivered by the laboratory chow fed to the rabbits came from carbohydrate sources.

- When the same studies were repeated in diabetic rabbits under conditions where insulin secretion was blocked by pharmacological drugs, atherosclerotic lesions did not appear, no matter how much cholesterol was added to the diet. Yet when the high-cholesterol diet was supplemented with insulin, atherosclerotic lesions reappeared in greater numbers throughout the vascular system. Within a few years, these findings were repeated in chickens and in dogs. It was insulin, not cholesterol, that seemed to make the difference.

Later studies showed that insulin enhances the transport of cholesterol and fats into the cells of the arterial wall and, furthermore, stimulates synthesis of cholesterol and fat in cells that line the arterial system. Robert Stout and John Vallance-Owen, the British diabetologist, suggested that "ingestion of large quantities of refined carbohydrate" leads first to hyperinsulinemia and insulin resistance and then to atherosclerosis and heart disease with fat deposited "in three sites, adipose tissue, liver and arterial wall."[1] Together with Russell Ross of the University of Washington, Stout showed that insulin also stimulates the proliferation of smooth muscle cells that line the interior of the arterial walls. This proliferative process also accompanies the thickening of the arterioles, which is characteristic of atherosclerosis and hypertension.

The insulin-atherosclerosis hypothesis appears to be the simplest explanation, not only for the close association of atherosclerosis with diabetes but also for the association of high carbohydrate diets with the accelerated onset of diabetes and aging. As Gary Taubes concluded in *Good Calories, Bad Calories*, "... anything that raises blood sugar ... will lead to more atherosclerosis and heart disease ... and an accelerated pace of physical degeneration." Indeed, evidence increasingly points to the conclusion that consuming refined carbohydrates causes not just diabetes and heart disease, but virtually all the degenerative disorders of the Metabolic Syndrome.

The Metbolic Syndrome, Free Radicals, and Oxidative Stress

Raising blood sugar levels may also increase the production of reactive oxygen species (oxygen free radicals) and advanced glycation end products (AGEs).

Oxygen free radicals are produced during intracellular oxidation of glucose in the Krebs Cycle. During the process of oxidation, electrons are attached to oxygen atoms in the mitochondria, transforming stable oxygen molecules into unstable oxygen molecules that react haphazardly with other molecules. This is called oxidative stress. It occurs in the presence of excess oxygen free radicals. The targets of these nonspecific oxidation events, including proteins and lipids, slowly deteriorate with loss of specific molecular functions.

The body has evolved strong anti-oxidant systems to regulate these potentially harmful molecular events. However, in the presence of high carbohydrate intake leading to rapid increases in blood sugar and insulin, excessive appearance of oxygen free radicals may lead to deleterious consequences (harmful metabolic reactions) within the cell environment. It is entirely possible, in fact, that insulin resistance represents an evolutionary development that limits the harmful effects of oxygen free radicals on cellular function.

Metabolic Syndrome, Protein Glycation, and Advanced Glycation End Products

The harmful effects of excess glucose oxidation on cellular function are compounded in the presence of protein glycation and advanced glycation end products (AGEs).

This story started in the mid 1980s when Anthony Cerami, at Rockefeller University, and Frank Bunn, at Harvard, independently recognized that hyperglycemia was associated with the formation of hemoglobin A1c through the non-specific process of protein glycation. Simply put, glycation occurs when sugars (glucose or fructose) attach to a protein in a manner that is independent of specific enzyme reactions. Enzymes are important in molecular and cellular functions because they ensure that structural changes conform to tightly regulated metabolic programs. When sugars attach to proteins by *non-enzymatic* mechanisms, haphazard, unregulated reactions, such as random crosslinking of proteins, may occur.

The process of glycation is reversible. If the concentration of blood sugars is lowered, the sugar may disengage from the protein. However, sustained levels of protein glycation can facilitate the cross-linking of glycated proteins into foreign structures, including non-specific heterodimers and hetero-oligomers. The crosslinking process occurs initially when two glycated proteins are covalently linked to each other, a process that permanently binds one protein to another. Theoretically, this pathological process may continue until it produces large aggregates of proteins, not unlike those observed in the neurofibrillary tangles of Alzheimer's disease. Because the process of glycation and crosslinking is random and haphazard, it can result in the formation of advanced glycation end products (AGEs), proteins that are brought together in unnatural combinations that may be viewed as foreign to the organism.

AGEs have been associated with both diabetic complications and aging. In diabetics, AGEs correlate with the severity of diabetic complications. They accumulate in the membranes of kidney cells, nerve endings, and in various compartments of the eye, including the lens, the cornea, and the retina. AGEs accumulate in arterial walls throughout the body, where they facilitate the oxidation of LDL particles in atherosclerotic lesions. They accumulate in skin, where the crosslinking of collagen leads to loss of elasticity and the accelerated aging of skin. AGEs also accumulate in other collagen-rich organs, including bone, cartilage, and tendons.

Wherever AGEs accumulate, they give rise to vascular lesions and nerve conduction disorders. When formed in the eye, they may lead to blindness. LDL is particularly susceptible to oxidation and glycation, and oxidized LDLs appear to be markedly elevated in both diabetics and nondiabetic patients with arteriosclerosis. Oxidized LDLs appear to have a longer half-life in the blood stream and to resist the normal mechanisms for cellular uptake and degradation. Finally, oxidized LDL are abundantly present in atherosclerotic lesions, where they may be responsible for the tissue degeneration and "stiffness" that appears in the organs and tissues of diabetics and other patients who experience accelerated aging.

Because the accumulation of AGEs over time is harmful to the normal function of cells during the aging process, the body has developed mechanisms to recognize, capture, and dispose of these unnatural structures. Atherosclerotic lesions, for example, attract macrophages and other inflammatory cells in an attempt to clear the body of unnatural molecules. However, inflammatory processes are known to greatly increase the concentration of oxygen free radicals that give rise to many of these unnatural molecules in the first place, thus compounding the process.

Like glycation, advanced glycation end products are exacerbated by high blood glucose and insulin levels. The vicious cycle that results from unnatural processes that stem from hyperglycemia, hyperinsulinemia, and insulin resistance serves as a blunt warning to avoid the overconsumption of carbohydrates and refined sugars that is one of the apparent causes of diseases associated with aging in civilized societies.

Metabolic Syndrome, Insulin-Like Growth Factor, and Cancer

Epidemiologists have suggested that 70–80% of all cancers could be prevented by appropriate changes in diet and lifestyle. Indeed, it now appears that more cancer may be caused by diet than by exposure to or ingestion of carcinogenic and pre-carcinogenic substances from the environment, with the exception of tobacco in lung cancer.

Early epidemiological studies led cancer researchers to conclude that there was a causal connection between increased consumption of refined carbohydrate and sugar and increases in the incidence of cancer. For example, as early as the 1970s, Richard Doll and Bruce Armstrong had recorded a strong correlation between sugar intake and the incidence of cancers, including colon, rectal, breast, ovarian, prostate, kidney, nervous system, and testicular cancer. Other researchers noted that the nations with the highest consumption of sugar also had the highest rates of mortality from certain kinds of cancer, while those nations with the lowest consumption of sugar had the lowest rates of mortality from the same cancers.

Researchers not only recognize a connection between insulin and cancer, they have also implicated insulin-like growth factors (IGF) in the process as well. Consider the following:

- Insulin-like growth factor (IGF) is secreted by the liver and by tissues and cells throughout the body. IGF is structurally similar to insulin and can mimic its effects in certain respects. For example, it can stimulate muscle cells to uptake glucose, although the effect is small compared to insulin.
- Growth hormone (GH) stimulates IGF secretion, which functions locally where concentrations are highest. However, most tissues require at least two growth factors to optimize growth (e.g., insulin and IGF).
- Nutritional health apparently mediates the effects of growth hormone, through IGF, on target cells and tissues. If dietary intake is insufficient, IGF levels remain low even though GH levels remain high. Add the necessary food, and IGF levels will increase, causing significant increases in growth of cells.
- Unlike insulin, which responds immediately to an increase in glucose in the bloodstream, IGF concentrations in the circulation change only slowly over days to weeks. Insulin has an affinity for both insulin receptors and IGF receptors in the cell membrane. If insulin levels are high enough, it will stimulate both insulin pathways and IGF pathways within target cells.

- Cellular receptors for both insulin and IGF are required for cancer-cell growth and proliferation. Down regulation in these receptors results in strong inhibition, if not total suppression, of tumor growth.
- Carrier proteins regulate the action of IGFs in the interstitial space between cells, because the complex is too large to enter the blood circulation. Insulin decreases the amounts of carrier proteins. Thus, anything that increases insulin levels will increase the availability of IGF to cells and increase IGF proliferation signals.
- Tumor cells overexpress IGF receptors (by two to three times), just as they over-express insulin receptors. IGF also inhibits or overrides the cell suicide program that prevents cancer cells from proliferating.

While the initial causes of cancer are not entirely known, IGFs and insulin are particularly important in stimulating the growth of cancer cells once they have achieved an adequate blood supply.

The levels of both insulin and IGFs can be modified by diet. To the extent that these levels are elevated by diet, the prevention and treatment of cancer may ultimately lie, in part, in the management of diet, including carbohydrate excess that characterizes the modern diet.

Metabolic Syndrome and Longevity

Genetic studies further suggest an inverse link between the Metabolic Syndrome and Longevity. Studies on mice, for example, have tested the connection between starvation diets and lifespan. Even mice that are genetically programmed to be obese can have their lives prolonged to normal and even above-normal lengths simply by reducing their caloric intake. The explanation for this seems to be, in part, that the restriction of the diet reduces the impacts of high blood sugar, insulin, insulin-like growth factors, glycation, and advanced glycation-end-products.

"Knock-out" studies on mice provide further support. When one of two IGF receptors was physically removed (knocked-out) from a test population, the mice lived 25% longer than a control group of normal mice. Other mice that were forced to consume massive amounts of food after insulin receptors were knocked out of their fat cells weighed 25% less and lived 20% longer than normal mice. According to C. Ronald Kahn, the senior author of the study, the knock-out mice were simply incapable of storing fat.

Long-lived cells and animals seem to share similar properties related to metabolic effects on fuel pathways. Reduced blood sugar, insulin, insulin resistance, and IGF levels lead to reductions in the levels of free radicals, decreases in glycation, and fewer advanced glycation end products, all of which may be involved in accelerated aging.

Genetic studies in yeast, worms, fruit flies, and mice have confirmed these hypotheses. In all four cases, mutations that confer extreme longevity on these organisms are mutations in the genes that control both insulin and IGF signaling.

For example, young worms (c. Elegans) will pass into "dauer," a state that is similar to hibernation in higher animals. The worms will enter into the dauer state only if they have insufficient food to survive. Genetic mutations that double the life span of adult worms affected both the dauer state as well as longevity. The mutation involved the worm equivalent of insulin-related genes in higher animals, including insulin and IGF. Similar mutants have been found in fruit flies that regulate conditions very similar to dauer and hibernation.

Longevity Hypotheses

As a result of the above studies, the current hypothesis is that lifelong reductions in blood sugar, insulin and IGF confer a longer and healthier life. The hypothetical factors that give rise to increased longevity may be summarized as follows:

- Insulin and IGF emerged as part of an evolutionary system to promote survival of the species when food is scarce. These hormone/growth factors regulate glucose metabolism, fat storage, and reproduction. IGF regulates cell division and growth. Insulin regulates metabolism by partitioning the food that we eat into calories for immediate consumption and calories to be stored for later use.
- When food is plentiful, activities in insulin and IGF pathways accelerate and stimulate the animal to grow, mature, and reproduce. When food is scarce, activities in these pathways favor long-term survival

over immediate reproduction. Thus as food declines, the animal begins to increase glycogen and fat stores and delay reproduction until food is restored.

- In the absence of food, the same pathways extend the lifespan of the organism, which increases the chances that reproduction may be successfully achieved later when the nutritional environment improves. This research supports the hypothesis that elevations of insulin and IGF will increase the risk of disease and shorten life.

It is reasonable to conclude that reductions in blood sugar, insulin, and IGF will confer a longer and healthier life on humans. At the same time, as Gary Taubes notes, "This research supports the hypothesis that elevations of insulin and IGF will increase the risk of disease and shorten life, and so any diet or lifestyle that elevates insulin and makes IGF more available to the cells and tissues is likely to be detrimental."

Summary

The Metabolic Syndrome represents a continuum of metabolic disorders that range from type 2 diabetes with accelerated heart disease, to patients with heart disease independent from diabetes to normal individuals suffering from accelerated aging. Numerous lines of evidence, including epidemiological studies and physiological studies, have supported high carbohydrate intake over a 10 to 20 year period as a major cause of metabolic disorders that are associated with this syndrome.

Further investigative studies with models of atherosclerosis, cancer and longevity are revealing. Insulin appears to be involved in fat transport into cells that line the arterial wall, free radical formation and oxidative stress, protein glycation, advanced glycation end products (AGE) and inflammatory processes that ultimately lead to atherosclerosis.

Metabolic studies indicate that proliferation and growth of cells involved in cancer depend on the simultaneous presence of both insulin and Insulin-like growth factor (IGF) that together signal the presence of energy resources that are required for cancer cell growth.

Longevity studies conducted on experimental models, including yeast, worms, fruit flies and mice, indicate that longevity is dependent on the scarcity of food, including carbohydrates that raise insulin and IGF levels. Reduced levels of insulin, IGF and blood sugar lead to increased longevity but reduced potential for reproduction. By contrast, the presence of rich food sources support pregnancy and growth in the newborn. These metabolic relationships, which are similar to those seen in hibernation of more primitive species, represent a powerful new concept in evolution.

These findings call attention to the deleterious effects of excess carbohydrate on metabolic processes that lead, in part, to the Metabolic Syndrome. However, because high carbohydrate diets are often low in protein, we need to analyze the other half of the equation, the pathological effects of deficiencies in amino acids, proteins and metabolic pathways on the development of the Metabolic Syndrome, which is associated with chronic degenerative diseases that lead to accelerated aging and early death. After we discuss the paradoxes of nutritional disease and obesity in advanced societies, the protein side of the equation will be revealed in the remaining chapters of this book.

Chapter 9

The Paradoxes of Nutritional Disease and Obesity in an Advanced Society

The Weight Gain Paradox

It is a great paradox that a country as wealthy as the United States has nutritional disease. Yet excess caloric diseases, including overweight conditions and obesity, abound in this country. The figures are staggering: 64.5% of adults are overweight, as are 32% of children between the ages of 6 and 19. Dieting is rampant, but most of those who lose weight gain it back. Many blame ever-increasing portion sizes and the proliferation of tasty, high-calorie foods that provide a day's worth of calories in a single meal.

America enjoys unparalleled wealth. Thanks to massive funding from the National Institutes of Health, we lead the world in scientific discovery and medical research. We have the most advanced medical practice in the world. We have recently sequenced the human genome and cracked the code for many of the genetic diseases that afflict the human race.

So, how is it that over the last 28 years, obesity has evolved into a major health problem? From 1960 through 1980, the obesity rate remained flat in this country. Then, between 1980 and 2000, the rate of obesity in the United States literally doubled. It is truly a paradox that the more we have discovered about health and diet, the less we seem to have learned.

This is a wealthy country with intelligent, appearance-conscious citizens. People have not chosen to become obese. So, how did this come about? Is it possible that, in spite of all we know, we really do not understand the causes of obesity? Could something be missing in our scientific and nutritional knowledge that prevents us from understand the paradox? Or could we have been deceiving ourselves all along about the causes of obesity?

Over-Abundance of Calories

Clearly, the most common cause of overweight disorders and obesity is the excess of calories consumed relative to the calories expended. Much of this imbalance can be attributed to a food industry that has developed an abundance of processed and convenience foods that are loaded with "empty calories." These foods excite the palate, but they are often devoid of essential nutrients and fail to fully satiate the appetite center. As a result, they tip the caloric scales toward unwanted weight, diseases associated with weight, and accelerated aging.

Seventy percent of the food in today's grocery stores and restaurants is processed food developed and packaged by the food industry. In as little as 100 years, the characteristics of the food supply have changed dramatically. In 1900, food was pulled from the ground, plucked from trees, harvested from grains, gathered as berries, fished from waters, milked from cows, or cooked after slaughter. Because humans evolved over millennia while eating fresh foods derived from an organic food chain that had itself evolved naturally over hundreds of millions of years, the metabolic processes found in plants, fish, birds, bees, animals, and humans existed in a balanced state of health and coexistence.

The twentieth-century food industry changed all that. The modern food industry developed sophisticated nationwide systems of food production and distribution. The evolutionary balance between diet and the food chain was disrupted overnight, as was the balance between calorie consumption and calorie expenditure. Factory-like agriculture methods, the domestication of wild animals and fowl, the introduction of crossbreeding techniques, the use of food chemicals, the development of cooking methods, the invention of refrigeration boxes, and the freezing of foods, all these transformed the methods of food processing.

The improvements in food quality have been questionable. Refrigeration and frozen foods have provided enormous advantages. Fertilizers have improved the yield of agriculture crops, and pesticides have improved crop yields and the shelf life of foods. At the same time, the industry has also introduced a myriad of chemicals into the food supply. The steroids and antibiotics that have been routinely administered to livestock have led to considerable controversy. Dwarfing all these in scale is the adulteration of food by food chemists intent on improving taste. For the first time in the history of life on earth, the caloric equation was upset in favor of food consumption predicated on taste, not nutrition. For reasons discussed below, the emergence of processed foods over the past 100 years has led to bulging waistlines and an epidemic of obesity in this country.

Processed Food

Over the past 50 years, the food industry enhanced the sugar and fat content of processed foods in order to appeal to taste buds on the tongue and in the oropharynx. These processed foods are now so common in grocery stores, health food stores, convenience stores, and fast food chains that many American consumers simply accept them as dietary staples.

Because processed foods are high in calories, low in nutritional value, and addictive, they pose a considerable threat to the sedentary societies of today's advanced world. Most people who consume these high-calorie processed foods filled with empty calories will gain excessive weight.

These processed foods violate a number of important nutritional principles. Chief among these are:

- Processed foods capture consumers in a "taste trap" of addictive, low-value, fattening foods
- Processed foods contain excessive amounts of sugar and complex carbohydrates
- Processed foods contain excessive amounts of fat
- The hydrogenated trans fats used in food fryers are particularly addictive and unhealthy. They are known to promote cardiovascular disease

Wholesale Grocery Stores

The problem of overeating has been accentuated by the proliferation of grocery superstores and wholesale clubs, such as Wal-Mart and Costco. The lower prices offered in these wholesale chains are reflected in the happy faces of dedicated customers. Oversized grocery carts, twice the size of regular carts, are brimming with oversized packages of food products, many of which are heavily processed. Unfortunately, the customers pushing these carts are considerably oversized themselves.

Restaurants Serve Super-Human Portions

Restaurants serve food portions that are excessive for sedentary consumers. Admittedly, it is difficult to cook for the masses when individuals vary widely in height, weight, gender, and age. Nevertheless, this phenomenon seems to cater to a national obsession with "bulk" and value for the dollar, in the context of a demand for profits, leading to ever-increasing prices for consumers.

Consider the businessmen who dine nightly in expensive restaurants on appetizers, main courses, salads, and bottles of wine, often one for each diner. In mild inebriation, diners often follow dinner with rich desserts and sweet after-dinner libations. Then, facing an early-morning workday, these businessmen retire to bed with full stomachs laden with food, wine, and dessert. This behavior typically leads to obesity and numerous gastrointestinal disorders, including gastroesophageal reflux disease, hiatus hernia, Barret's syndrome, and too frequently, esophageal cancer.

Similar eating styles exist at the other end of the economic spectrum. Blue-collar workers eat at fast food restaurants, where they consume huge portions of food and beverages loaded with sugar, carbohydrates, and hydrogenated fats. The French fries and onion rings are cooked in trans fat. Designed to maximize taste, these meals are fattening and addictive, so customers keep returning for more!

Four Nutritional Traps Lead to Obesity

Four nutritional traps lead to overweight disorders and obesity.

The Taste Trap

Processed foods with low-value, empty calories account for much of the increase in overweight conditions and obesity. These nutritional disorders play into the taste trap in which feedback mechanisms of nutrition and satiety are overwhelmed by the appeal of taste. Many of the processed foods can be found in fast food chains, convenience stores, and grocery stores. They include potato chips, cookies, cakes, pies, ice cream, popcorn, and other manufactured foods that have low nutritional value in spite of their high taste quotients.

Processed foods are low-value foods because they place excessive amounts of nutritionally harmful substances, such as simple sugars, in such consumables as fruit juices, soft drinks, and sweetened foods; starch-rich carbohydrates, including pastas, rice, potatoes, breads, muffins, and cereals; saturated fat in the form of cookies, cakes, pies, and fatty meats; and trans fat in fried and other fast foods as well as margarine.

These low-value processed foods were developed by the food industry to produce revenues and profits. The better the taste, the higher the sales. The "lip-smacking" taste associated with low-quality foods actually increases the concentration of taste buds that respond to these products in the oropharynx. The up-regulation of these taste buds, in effect, lends an addictive quality to the low-value foods, and this magnifies the nutritional disorders that result as a consequence.

The food industry initially believed it was improving food quality in the United States. However, by the late 20th century it became abundantly clear that these low-value processed foods had the opposite effect. They had become the major cause of obesity in the United States.

The Vanity Trap

Individuals with normal body weights in today's culture exhibit a different kind of nutritional disease that is disturbing in its own right. Out of vanity, many of these individuals try to avoid weight gain by restricting the kinds of food that they eat. Many highly educated professionals are found in this group.

Breakfast usually consists of a cup of coffee, frequently mixed with milk or cream, sugar or a sugar substitute, and either a bowl of cereal or pastries, such as a Danish, a muffin, a croissant, or a bagel. These foods lack protein. At the same time, the coffee is a mild gastric irritant that usually requires condiments to ingest, while the food items are rich in simple and complex carbohydrates and saturated fat. This breakfast is full of empty calories and does little to provide sustenance. It is also quite fattening even though the volume of food consumed is relatively small.

The "power lunch" may be somewhat more nutritious, but not by much. Sandwiches are heavy on the bread and mayonnaise, and the nutritional benefit of salads can be undone by gobs of rich dressings. Seeking to minimize the amount of food they eat, these dieters often replace proteins with carbohydrates.

The story gets worse. Disciplined individuals, intent on avoiding calories, may skip one or both of these meals or substitute a can of diet cola for lunch. The diet cola is laced with chemical sweeteners that double as gastrointestinal irritants. These dieters stay hungry all day long. Often they need to consume a powerbar with high glycerol content to get through the day.[1]

The longer they restrict the food they eat, the more famished these individuals become. Overcome by hunger pangs, they may turn to binge eating later in the evening. If these binges are composed of low-value, processed foods, these individuals will often experience, not weigh loss, but excessive weight gains.

The Food-Swing Trap

Pure sugars in the diet are rapidly absorbed into the body, where they rapidly increase the sugar levels in the blood circulation. This causes *hyperglycemia*, which is characterized by a "rush" of energy and increased clarity of thought. Naturally, this rush is pleasurable and desirable, at least for the moment.

However, as the level of simple sugars in the blood increases, signals are sent to the pancreas to secrete a correspondingly increased amount of insulin into the blood circulation. Increased insulin levels lead to the rapid transfer of sugar from the blood stream into cells of the organs and tissues. The result is often a rapid decrease in blood sugar and the concomitant symptoms of *hypoglycemia*. The symptoms of this debilitating metabolic state include headaches, dizziness, rapid heart rates, and a feeling of weakness, which may last for hours.

The Sedentary Trap

In fewer than 100 years, we have become the most sedentary people who have ever lived on earth.

Well-developed public and private transportation systems lessen the amount of exercise we get as we move around local communities. Washers, dryers, and dishwashers minimize the effort to keep house. Television has become the center of activity in the household, providing entertainment to ever-increasing numbers of immobile people. At work, we spend ever-greater amounts of time in front of the computer screens that control increasing amounts of the daily workload. Increasingly, children and teenagers watch movies and play video games instead of participating in sports or games on the playground.

Young and old, we are becoming a sedentary society that uses electronic devices in place of real-time human activities and human interactions. The changes are so dramatic across all age groups that it is no wonder body weights have climbed to unprecedented heights. All the indications suggest that this trend will continue, with no end in sight.

It is especially alarming to note the increasing sizes of pre-teen children. With energy to spare, children have normally been relatively undernourished during growth spurts. Today, overweight and obese children are so prevalent that clothes makers have begun manufacturing super-sized clothing for all these under-active kids.

At the same time as physical activities have become diminished, food intake has increased dramatically. This is particularly dangerous because increased food intake needs to be offset by increased physical activity. Instead, these two metabolic activities are moving in opposite directions at ever-increasing speeds.

Finally, the number of individuals and families who eat out in restaurants continues to rise. Fast food chains serve low-quality, addictive foods to increasing numbers of children and low-income families. Higher income families may eat foods with greater nutritional value in many such restaurants, but that advantage is offset by the huge portions served in such restaurants.

The Paradox of Age, Metabolic Health, and Body Weight

Age Changes the Potential for Unwanted Weight Gain

It is progressively more difficult to lose weight as we age. The reason is found in the fact that life is a process of growth and maturity. There are at least three distinct nutritional phases in life.

Phase 1: Growth, development & maturation (roughly through age 20)

Biology equips newborns of all species with robust metabolic systems that support growth, development, and maturation. These anabolic systems allow the newborn to grow and develop, first to avoid predators in the food chain and second to develop reproductive systems that allow the species to continue. Physiological systems support energy expenditures that often exceed food intake, normally culminating in vigorous, lean, healthy adults ready to assume the tasks of adulthood.

Phase 2: Adult life (roughly ages 21 through 50)

Adults in their twenties usually continue at the peak of health. Their hormonal systems are at their prime, and their health is optimal for promoting reproduction, a life force that requires robust health and stamina. Somewhere between the ages of 20 and 30, however, hormone levels begin a long slow decline. This is the beginning of aging and the onset of the accelerating process of catabolism. As hormonal systems and lifestyles change, nutritional systems begin to falter, and maintaining weight control becomes increasingly more difficult. To avoid the obesity associated with expanding waistlines, new dietary and nutritional parameters need to be put into place. Often, that involves the difficult challenge of changing accustomed habits and behaviors.

Phase 3: Menopause and Andropause (roughly age 51 and beyond)

Re-equilibrating nutritional health in the 30s and 40s is difficult. Achieving nutritional health in the 50s and beyond is immensely more difficult. This is because the robustness of health that supported reproductive life dramatically changes with menopause and andropause. During Phase 3, anabolic activities are progressively replaced by catabolic activities, and nutritional health becomes considerably more challenging.

The Weight Loss Paradox

Most investigators have assumed that the solution to obesity was rather simple: to lose weight, one needs only to eat less and exercise more. It is as simple as that. Furthermore, as promulgated by Ancel Keys, the McGovern Committee, and a long list of advisors over the past 60 years, anyone who is unsuccessful in losing weight is simply "undisciplined" and "poorly motivated."

However, the reality is that individuals who are obese or prone to gain unwanted weight, regardless of age, may eat no more than lean and healthy individuals. Often, they eat less!

Many individuals easily maintain their weight early in life and develop significant weight disorders later in life. In fact, most people, particularly as they age, have significantly greater difficulty in losing weight. A common complaint among older individuals is, "I am eating almost nothing and I cannot lose another pound!"

The Energy Conservation Paradox

We all remember the first law of thermodynamics: energy is neither created nor destroyed. Nutritionists have concluded from this that changes in body weight must be the result of differences between the calories taken in and the calories burned. Thus, the classic energy equation assumes that calories consumed and calories expended are independent variables. If that were so, then a change in energy balance would equate to the difference between calories taken in and the calories expended as shown below.

Change in Energy Stores = Energy Intake – Energy Expenditure

While this is an accurate means of expressing the overall equation of energy balance, many investigators have concluded from the first law of thermodynamics that there are no differences between calories: "a calorie is a calorie is a calorie." Investigators have further assumed that "energy intake" and "energy expenditure" are unrelated variables. Under constant energy expenditure, a reduction in energy intake should result in a reduction in energy stored as body fat. Accordingly, one of the axioms of weight loss has been calorie counting. Other things being equal, the thinking goes, people who consume fewer calories than they expend should lose weight.

The paradox in this case is that many individuals cannot seem to lose any weight, no matter how little they eat. Or if they do lose weight at the beginning of a diet, they gain it back over a very short period of time, sometimes even rebounding to a higher weight.

Fortunately, this particular paradox has now been largely solved.

Energy intake and energy expenditure are actually dependent variables. They are physiologically linked through cellular feedback and hormone mechanisms, so a change in one forces a change in the other. As seen in the studies of Jules Hirsch and Ethan Sims in chapter 1, energy intake clearly changes with energy expenditure, and vice versa.

Furthermore, high-fat/protein diets and high carbohydrate diets demonstrate different relationships between hunger, intake, exercise, and energy expenditure, because energy is expended differently through carbohydrate, fat, and protein pathways. Metabolic adaptations occur at every level. For example, when people diet to lose weight, their thyroids turn down hormone production and their metabolic rates slow down. When this happens, energy expenditure decreases, confounding our attempts to balance the energy equation. On the other hand, people will also increase their metabolic rates and energy expenditure when they consume a surplus of calories.

Energy storage is a complex interaction of opposing biological forces that are determined by both genetics and the environment. In *Good Calories, Bad Calories,* Gary Taubes discusses energy conservation and concludes that "The crucial factor is not how much is eaten—how many calories are consumed—or how much is expended, but how those nutrients or the energy they contain is ultimately distributed, how those calories are utilized and made available when needed. It is not [simply] the energy balance that is driving the system, but the distribution of that energy, the demand for energy at the cellular level."

The Exercise Paradox

Common Assumptions

It is often assumed that exercise is necessary for weight loss. Public health messages and weight-loss books abound in advice to engage in daily physical exercise, while personal trainers and exercise spas get wealthy counseling overweight people on the benefits of aerobic exercise. The USDA Dietary Guidelines recommend exercise and activity as a way to enhance weight loss while eating less. In spite of these exhortations, it is still difficult, and in some cases impossible, to persuade obese persons to engage in more physical activity. Age, too, is a factor. The more people age, the less active they become.

Scientific Evidence Short on the Benefits of Exercise

In 1960, even before the exercise craze, Alvan Feinstein examined the various obesity treatments in the *Journal of Chronic Diseases*. He concluded that "There has been ample demonstration that exercise is an ineffective method of increasing energy output, since it takes far too much activity to burn up enough calories for a significant weight loss."

In spite of Feinstein's conclusions, diet gurus like Jean Mayer and Jane Brody continued to claim that exercise was the key to weight loss. The public continued to listen. And researchers continued to be unable to confirm the exercise hypothesis. In 1973, for example, a Swedish investigator reported that after six months of exercise, his subjects were no lighter and no less fat than they were when the clinical trials began. Four years later, a group of 27 sedentary subjects in Denmark endured intensive training to run marathons. After 18 months of strenuous exercise, the average weight loss for 18 men was 5 pounds. The nine women lost no weight. In 2000, Finnish investigators reviewed a dozen clinical trials that tested the benefits of exercise on weight control or the prevention of "unhealthy weight gain." Depending on the group studied, their study led either to a decrease of 3.2 ounces per month in weight gained or regained or to an increase of 1.8 ounces.

As rewarding and healthful as exercise may be, there is no direct, linear relationship between exercise and weight loss. Part of this may be explained by the observed fact that people who exercise often eat more, and there are no guarantees that they will not consume more calories than they expend during their exercise. The relationship between exercise and weight loss is certainly much more complicated than it was once believed. As Julia Stern, of the University of California wrote, "when surveying the scientific literature on the treatment of obesity one cannot help but come away…underwhelmed by the minor contribution of exercise to most weight loss programs."

Potential Advantage of Exercise

This is not to say that exercise is not healthy. Even when viewed through the lens of weight control alone, exercise may be more beneficial in individuals who consume high-fat diets than those who consume high-carbohydrate diets. In the absence of carbohydrate intake and increased levels of insulin in the bloodstream, exercise increases lipoprotein lipase activity in muscle tissue, enhancing the oxidation of fatty acids after they have been absorbed into the muscles. Exercise will also burn more glucose, but carbohydrate-rich diets may lead to greater hunger that leads in turn to excessive intake of carbohydrate-rich foods, a process that may negate the beneficial effects of exercise.

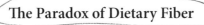

The Paradox of Dietary Fiber

While we are discussing paradoxes that impinge on weight control, this is a good time to address the role of dietary fiber in body health. This story parallels that of Denis Burkitt, a brilliant clinical investigator who began his career as a missionary surgeon in Uganda in 1947. Early in his career, he became well known for his studies on the fatal childhood cancer that came to be known as Burkitt's lymphoma, the first cancer to be linked to a viral cause. In the latter part of his career, he became the major proponent of dietary fiber as a way to combat the diseases of civilization, a position that supported the earlier work of Cleave described in chapter 2.

Burkett had established a network of 150 mostly missionary hospitals in rural Africa unaffected by industrialization. Burkitt and his colleague, Alec Walker, observed that "diets containing the natural amount of fiber are eaten and result in large, soft stools that traverse the intestine rapidly. By contrast, the refined low-fiber foods of the economically-developed countries produce small firm stools which pass through the gut very slowly" and lead to constipation.

Burkitt initially believed that low-fiber diets played a pivotal role in appendicitis, diverticulitis, and both benign and malignant tumors of the colon and rectum. Within two years, he had extended his hypothesis from these colonic diseases to all chronic diseases of civilization. However, Burkitt's fiber hypothesis was not supported by further studies. The results of the Women's Health Initiative, with 49,000 patients, published in 2006, confirmed that increasing the fiber in the diet by including more whole grains, fruits, and vegetables had no beneficial effects on colon cancer; nor did it prevent heart disease, breast cancer, or weight loss.

However, despite the negative findings of the WHI study, the final word is not in on dietary fiber, which represents the indigestible carbohydrates in vegetables, starches, and grains. Not only does fiber have beneficial effects on stool formation, regularity of bowel function, and cholesterol levels, but recent studies have indicated that dietary fiber can reduce the absorption of calories in the diet. Whereas 8% of dietary calories are normally passed unabsorbed into the stool, in one recent study the addition of insoluble fiber (roughage) increased the amount of unabsorbed calories to 25.6% over a 30-day period. Over the same period of time, experimental subjects lost an average of 8 pounds of body weight. Insoluble fiber may bind to digestive enzymes in the intestinal lumen and thereby slow the digestive process, limiting the number of calories absorbed into the body. Additional studies need to be performed on different types of insoluble fiber to understand further its role in limiting absorption of calories from the diet.

Summary

Over the past 50 years, while public policy has been misaligned with experimental fact, many dedicated investigators have spent considerable efforts investigating the molecular mechanisms that regulate food digestion and assimilation, as well as nutrient absorption, distribution, storage, and utilization. As a result, we now understand, to a much greater degree, the causal relationships that lead to obesity. Nevertheless, we have not yet put the whole puzzle together. Numerous paradoxes of weight gain and weight loss persist.

This chapter presents six paradoxes that concern overweight disorders and obesity. These include the weight gain paradox, that relates to the four nutritional traps leading to obesity, the weight loss paradox, that relates to selective protein deficiency syndrome, the energy conservation paradox, the paradoxical effects of age on body weight, the exercise paradox and the dietary fiber paradox.

While some of these paradoxes may now be explained, others remain problematic. The remaining chapters of this book will provide many of the missing pieces that will elucidate, to a greater extent, the role of "selective protein deficiency syndrome" in unwanted weight gain and resistance to weight loss efforts. We turn to this subject in the next chapter.

Part 4

Selective Protein Deficiency Syndrome and Weight Control

"It is one thing to know thoroughly and be able to teach well any given subject…, it is quite another thing to be able to take up that subject and by original work and investigation add to our stock of knowledge concerning it, or throw light upon the dark problems which may surround it."

– William Osler

Chapter 10

Selective Protein Deficiency Syndrome and Obesity

The Role of Protein Deficiency in Obesity

The four nutritional traps that lead to unwanted weight gains—the taste trap, the vanity trap, the food-swing trap, and the sedentary trap—are all characterized by deficiencies in protein relative to other food components. Such protein deficiency during fasting states and periods of carbohydrate ingestion may play an important role in the development of overweight conditions and obesity. Accordingly, addressing protein deficiency may be critical in the treatment of overweight conditions.

A detailed look at the consequences of protein deficiency will demonstrate why protein cannot be safely ignored in the diet.

Selective Protein Deficiency Syndrome

Healthy cells contain proteins that span the entire charge spectrum, from negative-charged proteins to positive-charged proteins. This may be easily demonstrated by spreading the proteins out on a two-dimension (2D) gel, as seen below in Figure 10-1 and earlier in chapter 3.

The light and dark triangles shown at the top of the gels, marked with negative and positive symbols, show the graded distribution of positive (dark) and negative (light) charges that reside in the proteins. Proteins at the far right in the 2D gel contain mostly positive-charged amino acids and few negative-charged amino acids. In contrast, proteins at the far left in the 2D gel contain mostly negative-charged amino acids and few positive-charged amino acids.

Figure 10-1A shows a 2D gel displaying, in schematic fashion, 10 proteins (round black spots) separated according to charge on the horizontal axis and size on the vertical axis. Each protein has a distinct, specific function that ensures the health of cells, organs, and tissues. Because the functions of proteins are complementary, the entire set of proteins are

Figures 10-1A, 10-1B, and 10-1C: Selective Protein Deficiency Syndrome

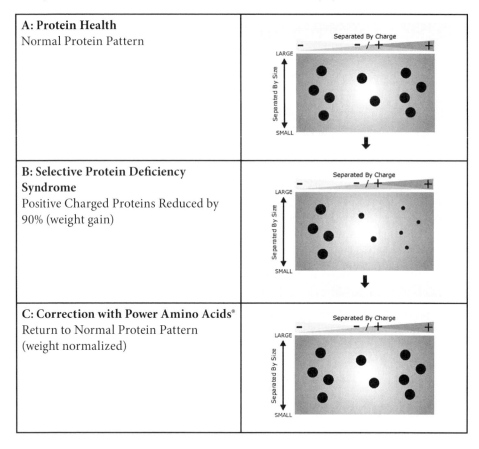

A: Protein Health Normal Protein Pattern	
B: Selective Protein Deficiency Syndrome Positive Charged Proteins Reduced by 90% (weight gain)	
C: Correction with Power Amino Acids® Return to Normal Protein Pattern (weight normalized)	

required to ensure protein health in a given organ or tissue. The pattern of protein expression[1] shown in Figure 10-1A represents a "healthy tissue." As explained in chapter 3 and here, the entire repertoire of proteins found in all the organs and tissues distributed throughout the human body are estimated at 20,000. However, the simplified pattern of 10 proteins shown in Figure 1 will suffice to illustrate the changes observed in positive-charged proteins in response to deficiencies in protein in the diet. In other words, a similar pattern of changes observed for the 10 proteins shown in Figure 1 can be expected to occur in the entire repertoire of 20,000 proteins distributed throughout the human body.

Under conditions of protein deficiency or partial protein deficiency, positive-charged proteins are initially affected more than negative-charged proteins, as seen in Figure 10-1B. In the example shown, the synthesis of negative-charged proteins continued, but the synthesis of positive-charged proteins was diminished to levels that were more than 90% lower than levels observed in health. Under these conditions of protein deficiency, positive-charged proteins showed up at levels that were lower than 10% of healthy levels. These changes in protein expression can be expected to result in serious impairments in cellular function. In fact, the impairments in protein expression may be expected to lead to impairments in metabolic pathways that result in serious disease states, including overweight disorders, high blood pressure, high cholesterol levels, and Type II diabetes, and even risk factors that lead to symptoms of premature aging.[2]

Amino acids provide the critical nutritional elements to correct the protein deficiency observed in Figure 10-1B. When the amino acid balance is restored, the pattern of protein expression returns to that observed in health seen in Figure 10-1C (compare Figure 10-1C to 10-1A).

How to Analyze "Proteins" on 2D Gels

The 2D gel shows the protein pattern observed for the sample studied. An investigator can determine three important pieces of information from proteins that are separated on 2D gels.

- Each separate spot represents a different protein. As a result, the number of proteins analyzed can be easily counted. For example, Figure 1A shows the separation of 10 proteins in this particular example
- Each protein has a unique position, expressed as a set of coordinates, in 2D gels. The coordinates, representing both the charge and size of the protein, allow the investigator to identify individual proteins between one gel and another
- Finally, the size of each spot varies according to the amount of the individual protein in the sample analyzed. If the amount of an individual protein increases, the corresponding protein spot becomes larger. Conversely, if the amount of protein decreases, the corresponding spot becomes smaller. Note that in Figure 10-1B, the spots for the positive-charged proteins are significantly decreased in size, indicating a deficiency of protein. Note also that in Figure 10-1C, the spot sizes for positive-charged proteins have been restored to those observed in the healthy sample depicted in Figure 10-1A

Figure 10-1 demonstrates schematically the pattern of proteins observed in health (Figure 10-1A), during protein deficiency (Figure 10-1B), and after correcting the protein deficiency with power amino acids (Figure 10-1C).

Background & History on 2D Gel Electrophoresis

In 1975, I invented the *two-dimensional gel electrophoresis* technique for separating proteins in humans and other higher animals. This procedure isolates proteins according to their surface charge in the first dimension, and according to their molecular size in the second dimension (see Figure 10-1). This new procedure enabled researchers, for the first time, to completely separate cellular proteins throughout the body. As mentioned before, the entire protein "repertoire" or "team" approximates 20,000 distinct proteins with separate functions that work together as part of the human proteome. In the pancreas, this procedure allowed the first detailed comparison of pancreatic digestive enzymes, including the iso-enzymes that digest protein, carbohydrate, and fat in the diet (the digestive proteome). It was a major scientific breakthrough, one that allowed my laboratory at the Rockefeller University and my colleagues in Europe to make seminal discoveries in pancreatic physiology, molecular biology, and cell biology over the ensuing 30 years. This method has been so successful that it is now used in scientific and medical laboratories throughout the world.

Role of Positive-charged and Negative-charged Proteins in Protein Health and Disease

In healthy individuals who have adequate protein substrates in the diet, each cell in the body is capable of synthesizing the full spectrum of proteins, including negative-charged and positive-charged proteins. Since each protein has a distinct function, cells that synthesize the entire set of proteins function at peak efficiency. We recognize this as the optimal state of nutritional and protein health and refer to this pattern later in the book as "supercharged" health.

Under conditions of protein deficiency, when essential, branched, and positively charged amino acids (which I refer to as *power amino acids*) are underrepresented, cell performance is limited, and the cells cannot produce the entire spectrum of proteins in adequate quantities. *Positive-charged proteins decrease the most drastically.*

The deficits in positive-charged proteins relative to negative-charged *proteins* can be attributed to dangerously low levels of positive-charged *amino acids* in the body. Positive-charged amino acids decline the most in the early stages of protein deficiency because mammals are incapable of synthesizing essential amino acids, including Lysine and Histidine, two of the three positive-charged amino acids[3].

In the absence or deficiency of positive-charged proteins, the body may continue to function but under greatly compromised circumstances. Under these conditions, we can survive, but the level of function, as measured by nutritional and protein health, is significantly compromised. For example, diverse physiological systems, including the cardiovascular, pulmonary, central nervous, immune, nutritional, reproductive, and other systems, can be expected to function inefficiently, unable to provide all the working protein units that the cells in organs need to be in a state of good health. When viewed in this perspective, it is easy to see that, during periods of protein deficiency, serious dysfunctions, including disease, may arise in inflammation, blood pressure, cholesterol metabolism, glucose metabolism, resistance to infectious organisms, weight control, and the like.

Protein Deficiency Leads to Fat Storage and Weight Gain

Poor nutrition leads to protein deficiency states that result in unwanted weight gain through the four nutritional traps associated with obesity, as discussed in Chapter 9.

Protein deficiency appears to lead to an imbalance between fat storage and fat metabolism. Under these conditions, fat storage exceeds fat metabolism, and fat pads increase without restraint. Protein deficiency also appears to lead to poor nutritional health and accelerated aging.

Power Amino Acids Correct Protein Deficiency, Poor Nutritional Health, and Overweight Conditions

Power amino acids are necessary to correct protein deficiency disorders. They are critical nutrients that the human body does not produce. These power amino acids enable the body to manufacture the full complement of cellular proteins, including both positive-charged and negative-charged proteins. In the presence of the full complement of proteins, the cell returns to a state of nutritional or protein health, a state that appears to reset metabolic pathways and balance the caloric equation.

Because of the benefits of power amino acids for protein health and the role of protein health in weight control, we conducted a weight-loss study to determine if power amino acids consumed as a supplemental health drink would induce significant weight loss and sustained weight control in obese subjects. This study allowed us to test the hypothesis that protein deficiency leads to unwanted weight gains and that treatment of these deficiencies with power amino acids leads to weight loss and sustained weight control in individuals with long-standing overweight disorders. The initial 3-month study commenced during the week of May 15, 2006 and extended through August 15, 2006[4].

We named this the "Factor4 Health Study" because power amino acids optimize the health of human subjects in four distinct ways that lead to supercharged health, as discussed in detail in later chapters. Thirty obese subjects entered the study. Twenty-six of these subjects completed the entire 3-month study. One subject had to be dropped from the statistical analysis because her weight exceeded the scale capacity.

Each of the subjects had suffered from chronic, refractory overweight and obese conditions for many years, most for more than 10 to 20 years. The majority of these subjects had tried popular diets and weight-loss medications with little long-term success. While they had been successful in losing a few pounds with each diet, they were unable to sustain weight loss due to a variety of reasons.

Results of the Weight Loss Study

Twenty four out of twenty-five subjects (96%) lost weight during the 3-month study, confirming our hypothesis that power amino acids were important factors in weight loss. At the end of this initial study, weight loss performance fell roughly into three groups:

- Modest weight loss (between 3 and 9 pounds)—thirteen subjects lost up to 9 pounds

- Moderate weight loss (between 10 and 19 pounds)—six subjects lost 10 to 19 pounds of weight
- Large-scale weight loss (between 20 and 29 pounds)—five subjects lost between 20 and 29 pounds

Because of the success of the 3-month study, we decided to determine whether a subgroup of subjects would continue to lose weight by remaining on the Factor4 Health regimen for longer periods of time. Thirteen subjects signed up to continue the weight-loss regimen for an additional 3-month period. Those subjects who lost moderate and significant amounts of weight showed steady, cumulative, and persistent weight loss over 6 months.

In order to be certain that weight loss subjects would continue to normalize their weight and avoid rebound to overweight conditions, eight of the subjects were studied for 12 months. Again, each of these subjects continued to lose weight and approached their weight loss goals.

The importance of power amino acids was validated by comparing the weight loss success under a regimen of power amino acids with weight loss achieved under four other popular weight loss plans, as shown in the table below. Weight loss from the Atkins, National Guidelines, Dean Ornish, and Zone diets was based on a 12-month study conducted on 612 subjects divided into four equal groups by unbiased observers and published in the *Journal of the American Medical Association* in March of 2007 as a separate study.

Table 10-1

DIET PLAN	WEIGHT LOSS
Power Amino Acids (12 months)	33 lbs
Power Amino Acids (6 months)	21 lbs
Atkins (12 months)	10 lbs
National Guidelines (12 months)	6 lbs
Dean Ornish (12 months)	5 lbs
Zone (12 months)	3.5 lbs

Final Results

Based on weekly measurements of body weight and body composition (percent body fat, fat pounds, lean body mass, total body water, and body mass index) in a group of 25 overweight adults (9 males and 16 females), the following positive effects were observed in those individuals treated with power amino acids:

- In the three-month study, 96% of subjects (24 out of 25 subjects) who followed the regimen of power amino acid lost weight over that period of time
- In a six-month study on 13 subjects, all of the subjects continued to lose additional weight during the 3 month extension
- During the twelve-month study, all 8 subjects continued to lose additional weight throughout the additional 6 month extension
- All subjects who lost weight also showed lower body mass indices at the end of the study period.

Conclusions of the Study

The majority of subjects had previous experience with weight-loss products and dietary regimens without sustained success. One subject could document unsuccessful experiences with more than 25 dietary regimens and 6 weight-loss medications over a 20-year period of time.

In contrast to the weight-loss products and dietary regimens that caused little or no sustained reductions in body weight, the power amino acid study documented significant, sustained, and persistent loss of weight with little change in dietary habits and little or no changes in exercise activity.

Follow-up Studies

In the two years since this initial pilot study, power amino acids have been used on more than 700 patients who suffered from overweight disorders and obesity. The more power amino acids they consumed throughout the day, the more weight loss they experienced. Individuals who committed themselves to this supplemental regimen and exercised portion control and selective meal replacements lost up to one pound every two days without experiencing excessive hunger. The long-term success of power amino acid regimens, moreover, suggests that this dietary supplement will continue to work for as long as subjects need to lose excess weight. The continued consumption of power amino acids promises to achieve long-term weight control as well as improved nutritional and metabolic health.

A General Theory of Nutrition

The discovery that protein deficiency can lead to specific changes in the expression of individual proteins in organs and tissues within a relatively short period of time measured in days or months has important implications for humans who suffer from overweight disorders and associated diseases as well.

Power amino acids have now been shown to induce significant weight loss and sustained weight control in humans with chronic refractory overweight disorders and obesity. These weight-loss results suggest that selective protein deficiency syndrome may play an important role in the development of overweight disorders in humans.

The demonstration of selective protein deficiency syndrome, a new discovery that appears to lead to an imbalance in metabolic pathways that store and burn fat, provides, for the first time, an explanation of the "weight loss paradox" that was discussed in Chapter 9. By correcting selective protein deficiency syndrome with power amino acids, it now becomes possible to solve this paradox and achieve meaningful weight loss in individuals who suffer from a wide spectrum of overweight disorders.

All told, these results suggest a general theory of nutrition and health that may explain why humans are prone to obesity and the other risk factors associated with the metabolic syndrome and accelerated aging. This theory will be defined in greater detail in the next chapter.

Summary

In this chapter we present startling findings, conducted on laboratory animals and analyzed by 2D gels, that link protein deficiency disorders with unwanted weight gain. These findings allowed us to develop the concept of "selective protein deficiency syndrome," which explains why people who are overweight often cannot lose weight, despite reducing food intake, a condition referred to as the "weight loss paradox" in Chapter 9. Because of the vulnerability in the food chain for the 9 essential amino acids, which mammals, including humans, do not produce, inadequate amounts of protein in the diet lead to rapid deficiencies in essential amino acids, positive-charged proteins and metabolic pathways that lead to unwanted weight gains and poor metabolic health. These experiments were conducted in laboratory animals.

We tested this hypothesis by treating a group of chronic refractory overweight humans with power amino acid supplements, which contain the complete set of essential amino acids and the three positive-charged amino acids, Arginine, Histidine and Lysine. In the first 3 months of the weight loss study, 96% of the subjects lost weight. When extended to 6 months and 12 months, subjects continued to lose significant amounts of additional weight. The weight loss performance observed with the power amino acid supplement, which led to the complete satisfaction of appetite, more than tripled the weight loss observed in four of the most popular diets studied over a 12 month period.

On the basis of these positive results, we have now treated more than 700 patients with power amino acids. Highly motivated subjects have lost up to 1 pound every 2 days or the equivalent of 20 pounds in 40 days. A number of subjects have lost 40, 50, 60 pounds or more. Based on these results we conclude that anyone can lose significant weight provided that they follow the instructions for weight loss that are included in chapters 12 and 13 of this book.

From the strength of these findings that demonstrated significant weight loss in the great majority of subjects, as well as significant improvements in metabolic health, we have formulated a general theory of nutrition that links power amino acid supplementation to metabolic health, weight control and revitalized youth. This theory is presented in detail in Chapter 11.

Chapter 11

General Theory of Nutrition, Metabolic Health and Weight Control

Primary Importance of Protein in the Diet

Protein is the primary and most important food staple of life for the following reasons:

- Protein is the only abundant food source that contains nitrogen
- Protein provides the building blocks—amino acids—for both the positive-charged and negative-charged proteins that lead to super-charged health
- Protein contains essential amino acids that mammals and humans cannot produce
- Protein can be utilized as fuel supplies for energy consumption, providing 4 calories per gram protein
- The amino acids contained in protein can be converted into glucose and fatty acids, providing the necessary substrates for carbohydrate and fat metabolism. In contrast, because carbohydrates and fatty acids lack nitrogen, they cannot be converted into amino acids

In these respects, protein is the primary food substrate for cellular metabolism and body health.

Proteins Provide the "Working Units" of Life

Proteins defy the second law of thermodynamics, which states that all matter moves from a state of higher energy to a state of lower energy. They act as working units, enzymes, that synthesize and degrade the organic molecules of life that are used to build, maintain, and repair the cells, organs, and tissues of the body. As enzymes, proteins establish metabolic pathways that synthesize and degrade the molecules of life, including proteins, lipids, and carbohydrates. Proteins are responsible for all the active processes of life, including metabolism, movement, and thought. Because many proteins function as enzymes that synthesize and degrade glycogen and fat, they also play a critical role in determining body weight.

Proteins Contain Essential and Nonessential Amino Acids

Proteins are made up of 20 different amino acids (see Table 11–1). In contrast to simple organisms like bacteria, yeast, and plants that can synthesize all 20 amino acids, mammals, including humans, can synthesize only eleven amino acids, those with simple synthetic pathways. Humans are completely dependent on dietary sources to obtain the other nine amino acids that are essential for life.

Table 11–1 lists all the amino acids according to their name, their three-letter code, their status as essential or nonessential dietary components, their charge, and their supplemental status as "power amino acids."

Table 11-1

Amino Acid	3-letter code	Dietary Status	Charge	Supplement Status
L-Lysine	Lys	Essential	Positive	Power
L-Arginine	Arg	Nonessential[1]	Positive	Power
L-Histidine	His	Essential	Positive	Power
L-Isoleucine	Ile	Essential		Power
L-Leucine	Leu	Essential		Power
L-Methionine	Met	Essential		Power
L-Phenylalanine	Phe	Essential		Power
L-Tryptophan	Trp	Essential		Power
L-Valine	Val	Essential		Power
L-Threonine	Thr	Essential		Power
L-Alanine	Ala	Nonessential		
L-Glycine	Gly	Nonessential[1]		
L-Aspartic acid	Asp	Nonessential	Negative	
L-Glutamic acid	Glu	Nonessential	Negative	
L-Proline	Pro	Nonessential[1]		
L-Serine	Ser	Nonessential		
L-Glutamine	Gln	Nonessential[1]		

L-Asparagine	Asn	Nonessential		
L-Cysteine	Cys	Nonessential[1]		
L-Tyrosine	Tyr	Nonessential[1]		

1. Arginine, as well as five other amino acids, is an essential amino acid in early childhood and possibly during growth spurts and illnesses.

Eleven of these amino acids are *nonessential*, which means that even though they are needed for health, they are synthesized by the body and are therefore not required in the diet. Under conditions of transient protein deficiency, during sleep or periods of fasting, the body can synthesize these amino acids. Therefore, these amino acids are generally of lesser concern.[1]

However, the nine *essential* amino acids cannot be synthesized by the body. Hence, they can be obtained only through the diet. During transient states of protein deficiency, these are the first amino acids to become depleted. Consequently, essential amino acids are of greater concern[1].

Power Amino Acids

Each of the amino acids shown as "essential" in the above chart is also listed as a *power amino acid*. Supplementation of these amino acids, many of which are hydrophobic, branched, or positive-charged, is critical during periods of protein deficiency. As a group, power amino acids rapidly correct protein deficiency disorders and generate positive-charged proteins in the body. As such, they are truly "powerful."

The term *power amino acids* was coined for the simple reason that many people without a scientific education in biology find it difficult to understand the differences between essential and non-essential amino acids. By calling these power amino acids, the *powerful* effects of these essential amino acids on human nutrition is emphasized, providing a more intuitive understanding of their importance to the lay community.

Even though it is often considered a nonessential amino acid, Arginine was included as a power amino acid for two reasons. First, Arginine plays a central role in the formation of nitric oxide, an important signaling molecule in cardiac health. Second, Arginine is also a positive-charged amino acid that is critical during early childhood and possibly during chronic degenerative disease later in life.

Three of the power amino acids are branched chain amino acids, which refers to the way the atoms are joined together in the molecule. The branched chain amino acids, Isoleucine, Leucine, and Valine, cannot be synthesized by humans. These three amino acids are rapidly lost during periods of protein deficiency.[2]

Protein Health

Lysine, Histidine, and Arginine are all positive-charged amino acids. Lysine and Histidine are both essential amino acids. As essential amino acids, Lysine and Histidine are rapidly lost during transient periods of protein deficiency. These three positive-charged amino acids are included in the group of power amino acids shown in the above table.

As positive-charged amino acids, Lysine, Histidine, and Arginine are essential for the synthesis of positive-charged proteins and enzymes. As shown in chapter 10, positive-charged proteins, many of which are enzymes, become rapidly depleted during transient periods of protein deficiency. With the disappearance of positive-charged proteins, we no longer demonstrate the full complement of proteins and enzymes that serve as "working units" in the cell. Without positive-charged proteins complementing negative-charged proteins, the body descends into a state of poor protein health and nutrition. Without the full spectrum of proteins, the team of proteins or "working units" becomes unbalanced, leading to impairments in metabolic pathways that adversely affect body metabolism.

The dietary studies that employed 2D gels provided the first insight into the consequences that rapidly follow conditions of protein deficiency. Within 12 days of lowering protein intake to between 0% and 10% of the diet compared to normal levels of 22%, experimental animals became grossly deficient in positive-charged proteins. Within this short period of time, positive-charged proteins decreased by up to 90–95%. In contrast, negative-charged proteins were unchanged. Under conditions of protein deficiency, the animals consumed larger quantities of carbohydrate that led to significant weight gains.

Because of the increased information seen on 2D gels that displayed individual proteins by their charge as well as their size, we were able to demonstrate, for the first time, how quickly the pattern of protein expression can change in simple dietary studies.

These studies underscore the critical importance of positive-charged amino acids in nutritional health. We now understand, beyond a shadow of a doubt, that positive-charged amino acids are more important in the food chain than negative-charged amino acids. This is the key that unlocks much of the conundrum about nutritional health and weight control. It all has to do with understanding the vulnerability of essential amino acids in the diet and the rapidity by which deficiencies in essential amino acids can lead to dramatic deficiencies in protein balance, metabolic pathways, and nutritional health. These discoveries underscore the importance of high-value (essential) amino acids and particularly high-value, positive-charged amino acids, which include Lysine, Histidine, and possibly Arginine as well.

Health Benefits of Power Amino Acids

By correcting deficiencies in essential amino acids, including positive-charged amino acids, the group of power amino acids can be expected to rebalance protein health, metabolic pathways, and nutritional health throughout the body. These corrective steps have powerful consequences for the entire body. It has now been demonstrated that power amino acids produce numerous positive effects on the health of organs and tissues in the body. A number of these effects are reviewed below, organized into four general categories or groups of health factors[3].

1. Metabolic Priming Factors

Power amino acids provide the anabolic building blocks for nutritional health, including strong bones, ligaments, and tendons to support our posture; healthy cartilage to articulate our joints; strong muscles to move our bodies; healthy organs to support the necessary metabolic activities required for life, and energy reserves to accomplish our goals on earth.

As building blocks, power amino acids prime the body by restoring nutritional health and balance in the eight major health systems in the body. These health systems are explained in detail in the next chapter.

2. Catabolic Releasing Factors

Power amino acids prevent the body from lapsing into catabolic states caused when starvation mechanisms activate cellular autophagy, a process by which cellular degradation occurs through self-digestion processes.

Catabolic reactions lead to food cravings, hunger pangs, and famished states that trigger eating binges. The correction of such states is critical for achieving nutritional health and weight control.

Catabolic states occur when daily starvation routines, including overnight fasting during sleep and daytime fasting through skipping meals, rapidly lead to selective protein deficiency syndrome, characterized by loss of positive-charged proteins in cells. During periods of protein deficiency, all of the cells in the body, and particularly the muscle cells, enter a state of catabolism. Catabolism leads to autodigestive states variously called "autophagy" or "endophagy." Within 15 minutes of the time that essential amino acids fall below physiological threshold levels in the blood stream, lysosomes are activated within the cytoplasm of all cells[4].

During this catabolic process, the cells digest—they literally eat—part of themselves to provide life-saving amino acids for the entire body.

Just as the whole body has a digestive system, the gastrointestinal tract, each cell contains numerous tiny structures called lysosomes, which serve as digestive organelles within individual cells. These lysosomes become activated during catabolic states. Activation of lysosomes allows these organelles to expand dramatically in size and ingest neighboring regions of the cell cytoplasm. At the same time, there is a dramatic increase in digestive enzymes that inhabit these organelles. This process of lysosomal activation and ingestion of cytoplasmic material represents a method by which the cell can breakdown its own protein structures to provide amino acids to the blood stream, which is important for survival of the organism.

Muscle cells suffer the most from autophagy, and this process gives rise to marked weakness or fatigue in individuals suffering from catabolic states in response to protein deficiency, whether partial or complete. Lysosomes may also attach to the cell membranes and secrete their contents of digestive enzymes into the extracellular medium. When this occurs, the degradative process that begins inside the cell may spread to extracellular sites and attack joints, connective tissue, blood vessels, and nerves in a process known as "exophagy."

Catabolic reactions lead to food cravings, hunger pangs, and famished states that trigger eating binges. The correction of catabolic states is critical for achieving nutritional health and weight control. Fortunately, catabolic states due to protein deficiency may be corrected by replenishing the body with power amino acids.

3. Appetite Suppressing Factors

Power amino acids show strong appetite suppression effects. Within 5 to 10 minutes of ingestion, individuals begin to notice feelings of comfort, satisfaction, and well-being that increase with time. These are the same feelings that individuals experience after eating a meal. Further research may determine that power amino acids actually provide the signals that communicate satiety to the appetite centers in the brain and digestive tract.

4. Fat-Burning Factors

Power amino acids treat obesity by correcting deficiencies in amino acids, proteins, and metabolic pathways, which rebalances body metabolism responsible for fat-storage and fat burning. The end result is that fat burning pathways appear to be re-established, leading to more effective weight loss. In short, this is the positive effect on body metabolism that allows individuals to conquer the "weight loss paradox" described in chapter 9.

These four factors appear to work together to increase anabolic health, decrease catabolic processes, and increase metabolic activities that not only burn calories, including fat, but also prevent excess food intake by curbing appetite and stimulating satiety in both the brain and digestive tract.

The health benefits of power amino acids, working through metabolic-priming, catabolic-releasing, appetite suppressing, and fat-burning factors, serve not only to supercharge health but to stimulate significant weight loss and sustained weight control.

Balance the Caloric Equation with Carbohydrate and Fat

Once protein health is established, hunger mechanisms will be controlled and metabolic pathways will shift from fat-storing to fat-burning pathways. When the body achieves supercharged-health, the "sweet-tooth" and the "fat-tooth" disappear. Once food cravings, hunger pangs, and famished states disappear, it is relatively easy to modify carbohydrate and fat intake to balance the caloric equation while maintaining a lean, attractive figure.

Importance of Amino Acids in the Food Chain

Mammals, including humans, are incapable of producing the complete set of amino acids that are required for life. By contrast, bacteria, yeast, and plants produce all twenty amino acids that are required for protein health. Accordingly, these lower organisms provide the initial source of essential amino acids required to sustain biological life on planet earth. The food chain is therefore crucial for moving essential nutrients, including essential amino acids, from lower organisms to higher animals. Because of these limitations in nutritional processes, humans are forever tethered to the food chain for their supply of the essential amino acids that are required for survival and optimal health.

In the food chain, humans eat high-protein foods like beef, chicken, and fish to obtain essential amino acids. However, cows, chickens, and fish also cannot produce these amino acids. Hence, the food chain is required to move essential amino acids from bacterial, yeast, and plant sources up to higher animals, including mammals and humans.

Power Amino Acids Rapidly Correct the Food Chain Gap

As shown by the 2D gel studies in the previous chapter, the vulnerability of the food chain, which may be described as the "food-chain gap," is first observed in the disappearance of positive-charged proteins that leads to poor nutritional, protein, and metabolic health.

While high-protein foods or protein supplements may satisfy the requirement for essential amino acids, power amino acids short-circuit the food chain the fastest. This is because amino acids are absorbed into the bloodstream within minutes. In contrast, protein supplements and high-protein foods require hours of digestion before their amino acids may be absorbed into the body. The difference in times of absorption, and therefore relief, may be observed in table 12-1.

We'll see in the next chapter that under conditions of amino acid deficiency, which is the primary determinant of hunger, power amino acids provide the quickest path to relief, followed by whey protein, casein protein, and high-protein foods, in that order.

Hypothesis Testing

As discussed in chapter 1, one of the ways to test the validity of a new hypothesis is to examine whether it provides new and improved explanations for previously unexplained findings. In a manner similar to that observed in chapter 1, we will examine this general theory of nutrition related to the importance of essential amino acids on nutritional health and longevity in isolated populations throughout the world that are celebrated for these traits.

Celebrity Food Cultures with Supercharged Health, Weight Control, and Longevity

Periodically, the American media have sought out locations in the world where the native inhabitants show superior longevity and health. The goal in these efforts has been to identify the dietary or lifestyle customs that lead to long, productive lives.

One place the media have repeatedly featured is Yuzuri Hara, a mountaintop village in Japan. Here, the inhabitants live well into their 80s and 90s, still working productively in their fields. They remain lean and well nourished and show very young looking skin. Reporter Connie Chung visited this village and produced a featured program on ABC television. Bill Sardi, the vitamin expert, visited Yuzuri Hara repeatedly to determine the secret by which these villagers retain youth. On one occasion, Mr. Sardi claimed that the youthful-looking skin was due to the ingestion of the hillside plant, Tamaji, which contains rich sources of hyaluronic acid.

However, the most likely cause of longevity in remote villages, whether they are on mountain tops in Japan and Russia or in the Savannahs of Africa, as inhabited by the Masai warriors, is fermented foods. In these remote locations, people have learned ,through trial and error, to preserve foods by fermentation. Since the fermentation process involves the use of bacterial or yeast cultures, these methods for preserving food also enrich the products with essential amino acids, which are produced in abundance by these primitive organisms.

For example, the traditional Japanese foods in these mountaintop villages include fermented vegetables, beans, and fish. The fermentation process is necessary to preserve food products during the winter season. Natto and miso are major soy-fermented products with different bacterial microbes. Umami is also rich in glutamate, which is generated through fermentation. During the production of sake, which is based on rice fermentation, an important by-product is rice curd, which serves as a rich food source for the traditional Japanese kitchen. Kasujiru is a miso soup version of rice curd. Fermented foods are rich in amino acids, including essential amino acids.

In addition to fermented foods, rice and soybeans have been the staple of the Japanese diet for centuries. Taken together, these two food products provide the full complement of amino acids, including essential amino acids.

In other parts of the world, notably in Russia and Turkey, fermented foods such as yoghurt are staples of nutrition. Yoghurt comes from milk fermented in lactobacilli, beneficial organisms that enrich these cultures with essential nutrients, including essential amino acids.

Although fermenting was initially used for its ability to preserve food, the bacteria and yeast in the fermentation process confer additional benefits to primitive societies. Rich fermentation cultures contain billions of probiotic, or "good," organisms. These generate essential and non-essential amino acids that are critical for prolonged life and good health.

According to the general theory of nutrition presented in this chapter, it is the fermentation process that facilitates the flow of essential amino acids along the food chain and results in the extraordinary longevity and health of these primitive societies. Thanks to television, these primitive societies have received celebrity status because they have achieved supercharged health and longevity through the primitive technologies they use to ferment foods.

But the story gets better, as the theory allows us to improve our understanding of the long-standing, symbiotic relationships between mammals and intestinal bacteria.

Fermentation Processes Provide Essential Amino Acids in the Gut Lumen of Larger Animals, Including Man

The role of fermentation cultures containing probiotic organisms in the health of higher organisms, including man, is powerfully illuminating. All mammals host trillions of probiotic bacteria, the so-called "good" bacteria, in their small intestine and colon. These bacterial cultures act as powerful generators of nutrients, including essential amino acids, that are necessary for optimal health in humans and animals.

Probiotic organisms are indispensable to human health. When these cultures are destroyed, by oral antibiotics, for example, the result is digestive disorders such as diarrhea and, more importantly, diminished protein health.

Cows offer another example of the importance of probiotic organisms in mammalian health. Unlike humans and other mammals, cows exist entirely on a vegetarian diet, primarily grass species grown in the fields. Like other vegetables, grass contains low levels of protein that are insufficient for building the enormous muscular architecture of these animals. As part of the evolutionary process, the stomachs in cows have developed four distinct compartments. The first of these compartments contains huge cultures of probiotic organisms that provide two essential functions for the host cow. The first is delivered by the enzyme called *cellulase*, which breaks down the specialized cellulose cell wall of the grass products (mammals, including humans, do not produce this enzyme as part of their repertoire of digestive enzymes). The second is fermentation, which greatly augments the production of amino acids, including both non-essential and essential amino acids. Without this multi-compart-mented stomach and the probiotic cultures that are contained therein, together with the probiotic cultures in the lower intestine, cows would not be able to survive.

Again it is the general theory of nutrition described here that adequately explains why mammals and humans have evolved tight links to fermentation processes in the intestinal lumen, which contain probiotic organisms ("good" bacteria) that act as generators of essential nutrients, including essential or power amino acids. However, it must be acknowledged that probiotic cultures of bacteria, while providing health benefits, do not fully compensate for the effects of food-chain gaps of essential amino acids. We know this from the dietary experiments that were performed with laboratory animals and analyzed with 2D gels in chapter 10. Despite normal flora (probiotic cultures) in their intestinal tracts, these animals still became rapidly depleted of essential and positive-charged amino acids.

The Importance of Power Amino Acids in Rebuilding the Body

Although it cannot be felt, the body is rebuilding itself every day[5]. This process involves rebuilding many of the proteins that allow the organs and tissues to function properly.

The state of youth, characterized by hormonal health, may be described as an anabolic state. This state leads to optimal health and performance. Webster's dictionary describes "ana" as upward, anew or increasing. "Anabolic" means increasing or constructive metabolism.

The state of aging, characterized by diminishing levels of hormones, may be described as a catabolic state. Webster's dictionary describes "cata" as down, away or decreasing. "Catabolic" means decreasing or destructive metabolism.

Supercharged health is characterized by anabolic processes associated with a complete set of proteins, balanced with both negative- and positive-charged proteins. In contrast, poor health appears to be characterized by catabolic processes associated with a relative absence of positive-charged proteins.

The critical element here is that catabolic states can be largely converted into anabolic states by supplementing the diet with power amino acids. Power amino acids may therefore turn destructive metabolic processes into constructive metabolic processes that convert poor nutritional health into supercharged health. Fortunately, it may also be able to transform much of the aging process into reinvigorated youth.

Furthermore, power amino acids have the added potential to supercharge anabolic health and youth on a sustained basis without fear of harmful side effects. Without power amino acids, the body will revert to a catabolic state associated with accelerated aging. However, the catabolic processes of aging may largely be converted into the anabolic processes of youth by including power amino acids in a dietary maintenance regimen.

Power Amino Acids and Protein Health Combat the Risk Factors Associated with Metabolic Syndrome

Power amino acids appear to have a number of beneficial effects on many of the risk factors that makeup Metabolic Syndrome, including the following:

- They promote significant weight loss and sustained weight control
- They appear to reduce both systolic and diastolic blood pressure
- They appear to reduce both LDL and triglycerides
- They appear to reduce blood sugar and therefore delay the onset of Type II diabetes

Efforts to achieve optimal weight control may also improve metabolic health and ameliorate some of the conditions associated with the Metabolic Syndrome[6]. With successful treatment of the risk factors that lead to the life-threatening diseases associated with Metabolic Syndrome, power amino acids can be expected to provide significant anti-aging benefits that increase anti-aging health and longevity in our society.

The General Theory of Nutrition Explains Many of the Paradoxes of Weight Loss Health

The general theory of nutrition described in this chapter links power amino acid supplementation to metabolic health and weight control. The theory explains how the early phases of protein deficiency, and more specifically selective protein deficiency syndrome, together with the harmful effects of excess carbohydrate, may lead to metabolic disturbances that result in overweight disorders.

The theory provides, for the first time, an adequate explanation for a number of paradoxes in weight loss health that confound our ability to achieve sustained weight control. By solving these paradoxes, the theory provides an improved rationale for stimulating weight loss and maintaining optimal weight levels. The general theory of nutrition thus provides a number of useful explanations related to body weight health that have not been adequately explained. These include the following:

The general theory of nutrition provides an explanation for the "weight loss paradox," which occurs when individuals drastically reduce their food intake but fail to lose weight. In this case the reductions in food intake may lead to selective protein deficiency syndrome, which impairs metabolic pathways that metabolize fat.

The general theory of nutrition provides an explanation for the "energy conservation paradox." The surprising findings here are that dietary changes result in changes in metabolic rates. Drastic reductions in food intake result in a slowing of metabolic rates; increases in food intake result in an acceleration of metabolic rates. These changes in metabolic rates may be related to changes in metabolic pathways that occur during the onset or resolution of selective protein deficiency syndrome.

The general theory of nutrition provides an explanation for the "exercise paradox." The surprising finding here is that while numerous studies have sought to demonstrate the beneficial effects of exercise on weight loss health, few, if any, of the studies could provide a clear-cut relationship between the two functions. Since these studies were conducted under varying dietary conditions, mostly in the presence of low-fat/protein diets, the onset of selective protein deficiency syndrome may have limited the metabolic pathways that promote fat metabolism. In addition, exercise leads to an increase in muscle mass, which may offset modest decreases in body fat that occur under these conditions.

The general theory of nutrition provides an explanation for the inefficiency of low-fat diets to reduce body fat. As described elsewhere in this book, more than 60 years of public health policy, initiated by Ancel Keys and others, promoted low-fat diets as effective weight loss measures. However, because fat follows protein in the normal diet, low fat diets are normally low in both fat and protein. Low fat/protein diets will activate selective protein deficiency syndrome, which may limit the metabolic pathways that burn fat.

Power Amino Acids and Protein Health Provide a Breakthrough Strategy in Weight Loss Health

The theory allows us to take a revolutionary step beyond the low fat/protein diets of public health policy and the high fat/protein diets of Dr. Atkins and other physicians to construct, for the first time, a low fat/carb diet that leads to significant weight loss without the drastic reductions in carbohydrate intake, as recommended by Dr. Atkins, or the starvation diets that lead to extreme hunger, as recommended by public policy proponents.

The "secret" that is revealed in this chapter, which presents a new theory on nutritional health, is that the use of a supplement of essential and positive-charged amino acids ("power amino acids") maintains anabolic/constructive health and, at the same time, achieves the feelings of comfort, satisfaction, and well-being that are associated with natural appetite suppression. Because of the power of amino acids to provide multiple benefits that correct deficiencies in amino acids, positive-charged proteins, metabolic pathways, and satiety that lead to improved weight loss health, the usage of the new term "power amino acids" is readily justified.

Summary

Based on the new discovery that the early indicator of protein deficiency is the loss of positive-charged proteins that lead to unbalanced metabolic pathways, a general theory of nutrition is presented that links this selective protein deficiency syndrome to the inability of higher animals including man to produce (synthesize) a group of 9 essential amino acids, which include hydrophobic, branched chain and positive-charged amino acids.

This theory provides a new understanding for how the early phases of protein deficiency, and more specifically selective protein deficiency syndrome, may lead to metabolic disturbances that result in the Metabolic Syndrome, which is associated with a number of chronic degenerative diseases, including overweight disorders and obesity, type 2 diabetes, cardiovascular disease, certain forms of cancer and other diseases that were originally classified as diseases of civilization.

The twin horns of selective protein deficiency syndrome and excessive carbohydrate intake, suffered over years, adequately explain the slow onset of chronic degenerative diseases that accelerate aging.

By closing the food chain gap with power amino acids that contain essential and positive-charged amino acids, protein health is restored and metabolic pathways rebalanced. The sum total of these corrections defined here as "supercharged health," provides the optimal state for the body to rebuild and repair the metabolic processes that lead to chronic disease and aging in the first place.

The general theory of nutrition provides, for the first time, an explanation for why individuals who are overweight have difficulty losing that weight when they reduce their food intake, described as the "weight loss paradox" in Chapter 9. Reduction in food intake results in selective protein deficiency syndrome and unbalanced metabolic pathways that prevent these individuals from burning fat under these conditions. The theory also resolves five other paradoxes related to overweight disorders and efforts to lose excess weight.

The general theory of nutrition links power amino acid supplementation to metabolic health and weight control. By providing this important new factor in body weight health, the theory allows us to take a revolutionary step beyond the high fat/protein diets of Dr. Atkins and other proponents and the low fat/protein diets of public health policy to achieve dramatic improvements in the success of weight loss health. For the first time we can construct a low fat/carb diet that leads to significant weight loss without starvation that leads to catabolic (destructive) health and extreme hunger. The theory teaches us that the use of a supplement of essential and positive-charged amino acids ("power amino acids") allows us to achieve anabolic (constructive) health while at the same time achieving the feelings of comfort, satisfaction and well-being that are associated with natural appetite suppression.

The general theory of nutrition also explains, for the first time, why higher animals, including humans are tethered to fermentation processes that occur within their gastrointestinal tracts and why isolated societies, scattered around the globe, enjoy supercharged health and extreme longevity based on a daily diet of fermented foods, which serve to partially close the food chain gap related to essential amino acids and optimal protein health.

As such, the concept of supercharged health provides important insights into a number of interrelated metabolic parameters that correct nutritional deficiencies in amino acids, proteins, metabolic pathways, body health and aging. It is therefore reasonable to assume that supercharged health will not only combat the Metabolic Syndrome, which leads to a broad spectrum of metabolic disorders, including obesity, but will lead to revitalized youth and anti-aging health as well.

The next two chapters will discuss, in detail, strategies for improving amino acid and protein health that leads to better weight control, metabolic health, and anti-aging health. The general theory of nutrition, as presented in this chapter, will figure prominently in achieving these goals.

Chapter 12

Strategies for Improving Protein Health

The Importance of Protein Health

The focus of this book is on the primary importance of protein health in achieving optimal body weight. This argument is largely new in the world of nutritional health. Nutritional scientists and physicians alike have generally assumed that protein health is not an issue in advanced societies.

However, the methods that nutritional scientists have traditionally used to assess protein health are insufficient to examine protein health on a protein-by-protein basis. This is why the 2D gel studies conducted on laboratory animals represented a breakthrough in scientific and medical research. This new technique allowed for the analysis of all proteins, on an individual basis, in any given tissue.

The high-resolution analysis of proteins spread on 2D gels provided the first diagnostic test for changes in protein patterns due to early protein deficiency. The dramatic decreases observed in the expression of positive-charged proteins within days of placing experimental animals on protein deficient diets suggested that protein health may indeed be more difficult to maintain than previously thought. Poor eating habits and age-related decreases in the efficiency of food digestion exacerbate this challenge to protein health.

From analyses of these studies, it became abundantly clear that the vulnerable shoulder of the food chain is represented by the poor efficiency with which positive-charged amino acids are moved up along the food chain. It also became equally clear that reversing the early forms of deficiencies in positive-charged amino acids and positive-charged proteins could effectively be achieved by providing the essential amino acids that are crucial to the diet of higher animals and humans.

Today, the fundamental question is how to ensure protein health in both advanced societies and underdeveloped cultures around the world. Can the vulnerabilities of the food chain be closed with high-protein foods obtained from the grocery store, high-protein supplements obtained from health food stores, or power amino acids that have only begun to emerge recently on a commercial scale?

How to Achieve Balanced Protein Health

Supplementation with High-protein Foods

Many people believe that the vulnerabilities of the food chain can be closed by simply increasing the amount of high-protein foods in the diet. After all, these are readily available in abundance in grocery chains throughout the advanced world.

Furthermore, a number of astute doctors have already called attention to the importance of high-protein foods in the diet. Although they were unaware of the "selective protein deficiency syndrome" that is reflected in the rapid loss of positive-charged proteins in the human proteome when dietary protein is limited, these doctors have correctly identified the critical need for adequate protein in the diet. A few of these doctors and their books are Dr. Robert Atkins, *The Atkins Diet;* Dr. Bill Wheeler, *The Gold Standard Protein;* Drs. Michael and Mary Dan Eads, *Protein Power;* Dr. Barry Sears, *The Zone Diet;* and Dr. Arthur Agatston, *The South Beach Diet.* Many people have lost weight on high-protein diets. Unfortunately, for reasons that are now becoming clear, much of the weight loss has been short-lived, and subjects have returned to the condition of overweight disorders.

There are a number of limitations to high-protein diets that are based on high-protein foods from the grocery store.

- High-protein foods contain secondary calories in the form of fat. This may explain, in part, why high-protein diets are ultimately unsuccessful. They contain too much saturated fat for long-term use. Because of these secondary calories, high-protein foods can be expected to lead to weight gain unless intense exercise routines are performed. This fact explains why overweight disorders often increase when dieters switch from fish to chicken and chicken to beef. Naturally, fish has less fat, chicken more, and beef the most
- High-protein foods are nearly always derived from muscle tissue in livestock, chicken, or fish. However, muscle tissue is enriched in negative-charged proteins and amino acids and diminished in positive-charged

proteins and amino acids. While negative-charged proteins do contain small quantities of positive-charged amino acids, the large amounts of negative-charged proteins that must be consumed to provide adequate quantities of positive-charged amino acids may exceed the parameters that balance the caloric equation

- High-protein foods are relatively expensive. In the farming industry, it is considerably more expensive to raise livestock than it is to grow vegetables. Livestock and meat products are more difficult to handle, more difficult to store, and, due to their perishable nature, more difficult to sell

- Most people who strive to eat a balanced diet are still deficient in protein. Economic factors run through the entire food industry. Not only are high-protein foods more expensive at the grocery store, but highly desirable cuts of meat that have fewer fat calories are significantly more expensive in both restaurants and stores. These economic factors explain why the wealthy often achieve greater weight control than the poor—they can afford to!

Given the abundance of processed foods, which are less expensive and more stable under prolonged storage conditions, it is becoming more difficult to maintain adequate protein intake through meat, poultry, and fish products. Although protein can be found in all varieties of vegetables, the protein content of most plants is insufficient to provide the daily minimum requirements for protein. Dairy products such as milk, cheese, and yoghurt provide an abundance of protein, but many adults have lost their taste for milk products, particularly those products that have been reduced in fat.

Supplementation with Purified Proteins

One way to avoid the secondary calories in high-protein foods is to supplement the diet with protein shakes. Four commercial proteins are generally available in health food stores. These are made from whey, casein, egg white, and soy. Supplementation of the diet with protein shakes can enhance protein intake to levels recommended by the USDA.

However, there are limitations to protein powders in closing the food chain gap.

- It takes significant time for proteins to be digested in the GI tract so that the amino acids can be absorbed into the bloodstream. Generally, whey protein requires about 2 hours for digestion. Casein requires about 8 hours. Egg white and soy require intermediate times. Because of the time required for digestion, the absorption of amino acids occurs even more slowly, and amino acid levels in the bloodstream may seldom reach thresholds that achieve appetite suppression
- All four protein supplements are enriched in negative-charged proteins and amino acids and diminished in positive-charged proteins and amino acids. It appears that vulnerabilities in the food chain, including deficiencies in hydrophobic, branched-chain, and positive-charged amino acids, restrict the amounts of proteins that can be produced in nature. Only negative-charged proteins may be produced in great abundance in nature. In spite of the considerable commercial utility of whey, casein, egg white, and soy proteins, these commercial proteins are lacking in the positive-charged amino acids that are crucial for rapidly closing the vulnerabilities of the food chain
- Because they seldom increase amino acid levels in the bloodstream to the threshold levels required to suppress appetite, protein shakes may well lead to weight gain unless intense exercise routines are employed

Protein supplementation in the diet with protein powders and shakes is an excellent way to achieve the minimal daily requirements for protein in the diet. And protein supplementation leads to better nutrition and health. However, in the absence of intense exercise routines, it has not been possible to show significant weight loss with protein powder supplementation alone.

Supplementation with Power Amino Acids
Supplementation of the diet with power amino acids avoids the limitations of both high-protein foods and protein shakes and provides a number of additional benefits:

- Power amino acid supplements avoid the problem of fat calories
- Power amino acid supplements are enriched in hydrophobic, branched-chain, and positive-charged amino acids that correct the

vulnerabilities in the food chain. These vulnerabilities are closed within minutes instead of the hours required by protein supplements and high-protein foods

- Power amino acid supplements help to meet the minimum daily requirements for protein in the diet in a way that better addresses the limitations of positive-charged amino acids in the diet
- Power amino acid supplements are absorbed quickly into the bloodstream and therefore lead to rapid appetite suppression
- Power amino acid supplements cost no more than protein supplements, and they are considerably less expensive than high-protein foods in grocery stores and restaurants

Comparison of Absorption Times for Power Amino Acids, Protein Shakes, and High Protein Foods

While high-protein foods or protein supplements may satisfy the requirements for essential amino acids, the availability of power amino acids short-circuits the food chain the fastest. This is because amino acids are absorbed into the bloodstream within a few minutes. Protein supplements require digestion before their amino acids may be absorbed. High-protein foods require additional periods of time for digestion and absorption. The difference may be observed in the table shown below.

Table 12-1

Source of essential amino acids	Time of absorption into the bloodstream
Power amino acids supplements	5 to 10 minutes
Whey protein	2 hours[1]
Casein protein	8 hours[1]
High-protein foods	Up to 15 hours[2]

[1] Data obtained from Protient, Inc.

[2] Data from *Experiments and Observations on Gastric Juice and the Physiology of Digestion* by William Beaumont, M.D., Surgeon in the U.S. Army

In conclusion, under conditions of amino acid and protein deficiency, which are the primary determinant of hunger, power amino acids provide the quickest path to relief, followed by whey protein, casein protein, and high-protein foods, in that order.

The Importance of Power Amino Acids
for the Four Cornerstones of Supercharged Health

There are four cornerstones of supercharged health: body weight control, metabolic health, youth revitalization, and anti-aging health. Amino acids, and particularly power amino acids, are integral to the integrity of these cornerstones. Over 700 patients have now taken power amino acids formulated into a proprietary health powder and added to water, soymilk, or low-fat milk. Numerous benefits have been recorded. These benefits are discussed below in relationship to the four cornerstones of supercharged health, which together may be defined as the highest level of health achieved through dietary means.

Cornerstone 1: Body Weight Control

The great majority of subjects reported significant energy gains and weight loss. Within 1–2 weeks of taking power amino acids, they claimed their energy levels had noticeably increased and remained increased as long as they continued taking these supplements. Because of their elevated energy levels, their physical activity increased naturally without training sessions or exercise classes.

As part of the changes observed in energy pathways, power amino acids activate the switch that converts fat-storage pathways to fat-burning pathways. This shift in metabolic pathways facilitates the burning of fat and disables the metabolic states that previously resisted weight loss, referred to as the "weight loss paradox" in chapter 9. They appear to activate the metabolic switches that increase the metabolism of fat and thereby combat the four nutritional traps that lead to overweight disorders and obesity.

Power amino acids reverse the catabolic activities that occur during transient periods of protein deficiency at the molecular and cellular levels. By releasing these catabolic states, power amino acids block food cravings, hunger pangs, and the famished states that lead to eating binges.

Power amino acids provide essential nutrients that satisfy the digestive system as well as the appetite centers in the brain. These nutrients reduce the desire for low-value foods that contain empty calories and lead to the food addictions associated with poor nutritional health.

Power amino acids enable consumers to make positive lifestyle changes that lead to accelerated weight loss.

As fat deposits decrease and lean body mass—muscle—increases, body tone shows noticeable improvements in firmness, even without exercise. At the same time, increased muscular strength allows the entire skeletal system to function better during daily activities, household chores, and stress-filled lives. Increased body strength improves posture and body coordination during walking, running, and other athletic activities. Improved physical and nutritional health restores the desire for exercise and sporting activities and improves performance in these activities as well[1].

Cornerstone 2: Metabolic Health

In addition to weight loss and sustained weight control, numerous additional beneficial effects were seen in metabolic health throughout the body. These results are presented here in table format according to eight major health systems that patients easily recognize. In addition, the beneficial effects, as measured by questionnaires and follow-up interviews, have been further qualified according to strength of validation by four criteria, including demonstration in published clinical trials for similar ingredients, demonstration according to testimonials, prediction with supporting evidence in the literature, and prediction based on general knowledge of science and medicine.

Table 12-2

Health System	Effects of the Factor4 Regimen
1 Body weight and energy health	Fat loss in extremities[2,4] Fat loss in central torso[2,4] Decreased total body weight[2,4] Increased pep & energy[2,4] Increased physical activity & exercise[2,4] Increased lean muscle mass[2,4] Enhanced muscle strength[2,4] Enhanced muscle relaxation[2]
2 Beauty health	Skin color, texture, moisture & health improved[2] Hair becomes smoother, thicker & healthier and grows faster[2] Nails increase in color, strength, and radiance and grow faster[2]

3 Mental balance/health	Clarity of thought improved[2] Memory improved[2,4] Mood swings stabilized[2] Stress levels reduced[2] Relief from depression[2] Relief from anxiety attacks[2] Relief from anger, rage and aggression[2] Enhanced sleep[2,3]
4 Digestive health	Taste adapts to high-value foods[2] Appetite satisfied more quickly[2] Calming effect on stomach[2] Decreased acid reflux & heart burn[2] Increased regularity of bowel movements[2]
5 Cardiovascular health	Blood pressure reduced with weight loss[1] Cholesterol levels reduced with weight loss[1] Blood sugar levels reduced[1] Type 2 diabetes reduced with weight loss[1] Metabolic Syndrome combated[2]
6 Immune health	Increased natural resistance to viruses[2] Increased natural resistance to bacteria[2] Increased natural resistance to fungi[2] Decreased free radicals[4] Decreased non-specific inflammation[4] Decreased C-reactive protein[4]
7 Reproductive and sexual health	Increased sexual desire[2] Increased erectile function[2] Increased sexual activity[2] Increased ejaculate volume[2]
8 Aging health	Decrease in tired, weak feelings[2] Increase in pep, energy & activity[2] Increase in comfort, satisfaction & well-being[2] Decreased functional age[2] Increased performance during aging[2]

1. Demonstrated in published clinical trials

2. Demonstrated in testimonials

3. Predicted with supporting evidence in literature

4. Predicted

Cornerstone 3: Youth Revitalization

Among the numerous positive benefits observed with power amino acids are anabolic processes that reclaim many of the characteristics associated with youth. These are discernable in energy levels, endurance, athletic performance, and desire for a more active lifestyle. The great majority of subjects experienced significant increases in pep, energy, activity, stamina, and endurance. Within 6 to 12 months of power amino acid supplementation, the effects were noticeable enough that many subjects believed that their "functional age" had been reduced by up to 10–20 years.

Cornerstone 4: Anti-Aging Health

Subjects reported losing the tired, sluggish feelings of advancing age, gaining confidence, and increasing their quality of life with feelings of comfort, satisfaction, and well-being. One older individual approaching 60 decreased his triathlon time by more than 10 minutes and decreased his recovery time from 24 to 15 hours. As a consequence of the increases in nutritional, metabolic, and anti-aging health, the catabolic processes associated with aging may be reduced, along with many of the risk factors and chronic degenerative diseases associated the Metabolic Syndrome that lead to accelerated aging and early death. As a result of these positive benefits, many older subjects compared themselves favorably to their age-mates in quality of life that relates to metabolic health and physical beauty.

Summary

Amino acid and protein health appear to be central components in improving weight control, metabolic health, and anti-aging health. While high-protein foods and protein supplements may improve protein health, there are distinct limitations in both of these nutritional strategies. In contrast, supplementation with power amino acids appears to be the most effective vehicle for rapidly improving the four cornerstones of health—weight control, metabolic health, youth revitalization, and anti-aging health—that lead to increased longevity and improved quality of life.

This chapter explains in detail why power amino acids are superior to high-protein foods and protein shakes in achieving the heretofore elusive goals of weight loss health that restores the body to a more youthful physique and improved metabolic health that combats the chronic degenerative diseases that often result in accelerated aging.

The next chapter will provide practical advice on what changes need to be made in the diet and how to use power amino acids to rapidly achieve supercharged health that leads to longevity characterized by optimal health.

Part 5

Dietary Health and Human Destiny

"Our food should be our medicine. Our medicine should be our food."

– Hippocrates

Chapter 13

Achieving Successful Weight Control

Dieting in America

According to MarketData, a market research company in Tampa, Florida, 72 million people, or approximately one quarter of the population, are normally engaged in dieting in the U.S. at any given time. Forty-four million (62%) are women and 28 million (38%) are men. In 2007, the diet industry was estimated at $58.7 billion.

Although diets to stimulate weight loss have been popular for centuries, they are less effective than generally believed for two main reasons:

- Popular diets drain the body of essential nutrients.
- Popular diets break down muscle tissue and body health through catabolic (destructive) reactions.

Weight Loss Meal Programs

Weight-loss meal programs have become popular for people suffering from overweight disorders and obesity. Designed by professional nutritionists, these meals may remove excess calories from the diet. In addition, meal programs are convenient for senior citizens who are unable to perform the grocery shopping and meal preparation efforts that result in healthy eating habits. However, meal programs may be insufficient to rid the body of excess unwanted fat without causing nutritional deficiencies.

Weight Loss Drugs

The major weight loss drugs that are sold or prescribed in America are listed in the table on the following page.

Phentermine, Phendimetrazine, and Diethylproprion lead to nervous agitation resulting in uncontrolled "jitters." So do neutraceutical or OTC drugs, including Caffeine, Guarana, and Theophylline. Consumer groups requested that Sibutramine be pulled from the market because of strokes and heart attacks. Orlistat, Meridian, and its OTC counterpart,

171

Table 13-1: Prescription Drugs

Drug Name	Drug action	Side effects
Phentermine (Adipex, Ionamin, Pro Fast)	The "Phen" half of Fen-Phen combination, now banned by the FDA, suppresses appetite through an amphetamine-like stimulation of the central nervous system.	• Nervous agitation • Elevated blood pressure • Potential dependency • Pulmonary hypertension is a rare side effect
Phendimetrazine (Adipost, Bontril, Phendiet)	Appetite suppressant & metabolic stimulant similar to Phentermine highly controlled because of a greater potential for abuse	• Nervous agitation • Elevated blood pressure • Potential dependency • Pulmonary hypertension
Diethylpropion (Tenuate, Tenuate dospan)	Similar to Phentermine and Phendimetrazine	• Nervous agitation • Elevated blood pressure • Potential dependency • Pulmonary hypertension
Sibutramine (Meridia)	Appetite suppressant working through a different mechanism	• Risk of a significant increase in blood pressure • Not for use in cardio-vascular diseases
Orlistat (Xenical)	Blocks the absorption of ingested fat	• Bloating, cramping, diarrhea & gas
Meridian (Sibutramine)	Blocks the absorption of ingested fat	• Bloating, cramping, diarrhea & gas

Table 13-2: Over-the-Counter (OTC) Drugs

Category	Drug action	Side effects
Lipase inhibitors Alli®	Drug inhibits the action of lipase in digesting dietary fat	• Bloating, cramping, diarrhea and gas
Amylase inhibitors Phaseolus (White bean extract)	Drug inhibits the action of amylase in digesting carbohydrate	• Bloating, cramping & gas
Stimulants (Caffeine, Theophylline, Guarana)	Metabolic stimulants in coffee and tea	• Nervous agitation • Elevated blood pressure • Potential dependency
Stomach expanding fibers (Glucomannans)	Glucomannan fibers expand by absorbing fluid in the stomach	• Bloating & loss of essential nutrients
Ephedra (Ma Huang) (FDA has declared this drug Illegal)	Metabolic stimulant	• Nervous agitation • Elevated blood pressure Reported deaths

Alli®, inhibit fat digestion and absorption but cause significant bloating, cramping, diarrhea, and gas and may lead to embarrassing gastrointestinal events. Drugs that inhibit carbohydrate digestion and absorption may lead to bloating, cramping, and gas. Many doctors believe that the harmful side effects of prescription and OTC weight loss drugs outweigh their potential benefits.

Appetite suppressants such as cocaine and methamphetamine are illegal, as is Ephedra (Ma Huang). Metabolic enhancers as well as illegal substances may further cause bodily harm, including death, and may accelerate aging as well. Fiber supplements decrease the digestive process in the intestinal tract, which may lead to nutritional deficiencies.

The bottom line is that all popular diets, meal programs, and weight-loss products have undesirable side effects, among which is the loss of essential nutrients, including vitamins, minerals, micronutrients, essential amino acids, and positive-charged proteins from the body.

Lose Weight and Improve Health at the Same Time

The secret to successfully controlling body weight and living a healthier life may be adding something to—rather than subtracting something from—the daily diet. As described in this book, the addition of power amino acids to the diet corrects the age- and diet-related deficiencies in amino acids, positive-charged proteins, and metabolic pathways that lead to poor nutritional health, overweight disorders, chronic degenerative disease, and accelerated aging.

A Factor4 regimen of power amino acids can help people reach their weight loss goals while maintaining optimal body health with or without popular diets, meal programs, or weight loss drugs for the following reasons. It:

- is complementary to other diet plans because it rebuilds the body with power amino acids, the essential ingredients for supercharged health
- corrects the "selective protein deficiency syndrome" that leads to overweight disorders and obesity in the first place
- suppresses appetite blocking food cravings, hunger pangs, famished states, and eating binges

- inhibits the desire for refined sugars and starch-rich foods that increase appetite and provide "empty calories" to the body
- improves metabolic health in the 8 major health systems of the body
- revitalizes youthfulness with pep, energy, activity, stamina, endurance, and performance
- increases anti-aging health with improved "quality of life," including greater feelings of comfort, satisfaction, and well-being
- provides supercharged protein health, converting many of the catabolic reactions of aging to the anabolic processes of youth
- resets metabolic pathways from fat storage to fat burning
- uses natural processes to rebalance the caloric equation and achieve weight loss health

The remainder of this chapter will describe how power amino acids may be used to achieve supercharged health that leads to loss of excess weight and sustained weight control. It will also provide practical advice on other changes that need to be made in the diet to achieve optimal body weight and anti-aging health without counting calories or points. Each of the recommendations for improved body weight and health derive from the general theory of nutrition, discussed in Chapters 11 and 12, that leads to metabolic health, weight control, revitalized youth, and anti-aging health.

How did all this develop in such a short period of time? Based on our earlier studies of protein health, we formulated, in 2005, a health powder that contains power amino acids, protein, vitamins, minerals, and micronutrients. The combination of amino acids and protein reserves was intended to ensure that amino acids were delivered to the bloodstream in two waves. The first wave would come from the rapid uptake of power amino acids within minutes of ingesting the formula. The second wave would result from the reserve of amino acids absorbed into the body after the digestion of the protein contained in the formula.

We called this formulation Factor4 Weight Control, or Factor4 for short, because it contained four groups of essential ingredients. To test the efficacy of power amino acids to address weight loss, we administered the formulation to more than 700 patients. The results have been dramatically positive, producing four reported benefits that promise significant weight loss and sustained weight control.

Benefit 1: Power Nutrition and Supercharged Health

Factor4 stimulated anabolic pathways ("constructive" processes) that lead to weight loss and sustained weight control. At the same time, it inhibited catabolic pathways ("destructive" processes) that lead to chronic degenerative disease and accelerated aging. The great majority of participants reported significant weight loss as well as improvements in metabolic health parameters throughout the body. Overall, they felt younger and healthier and experienced an improved quality of life.

Benefit 2: Appetite Suppression

Participants immediately noticed that the Factor4 regimen suppressed appetite, abolishing food cravings, hunger pangs, and famished states that led to eating binges. In place of cravings, they reported feelings of "comfort, satisfaction, and well-being" within minutes of consuming the Factor4 regimen. Many subjects were surprised at how quickly their "sweet tooth" and "fat tooth" disappeared. These changes in desire and taste diminished their cravings for snacks and meals loaded with refined sugars and high-density carbohydrates.

Benefit 3: Increased Energy

Within several weeks of starting the Factor4 program, subjects noticed that they had developed more "pep, energy, activity, stamina, and endurance." Many were surprised at their increased performance in daily work, household chores, exercise routines, and athletic performance. Increased body energy and strength implied that significant changes had occurred in metabolic pathways throughout the body. Changes in body metabolism also increased muscle tissue and decreased body fat. Since muscle tissue is the most important organ for burning off body fat, these two processes appear to work together to reset body weight and energy metabolism.

Benefit 4: Loss of Body Fat

Up to 96% of individuals who followed the program lost weight while taking the Factor4 regimen of power amino acids and other essential nutrients. Highly motivated subjects lost up to 1 pound every 2 days. A number of subjects lost 40, 50 and 60 pounds. Since weight loss was the primary benefit participants were seeking, the program achieved the measurable outcomes that subjects sought.

Weight Loss Takes Time

It is important to remember that it takes years to gain excess body weight. Consequently, dieters should understand that it takes time to lose those excess pounds and achieve the healthy, youthful physique that they seek.

In our experience with the Factor4 regimen of power amino acids, the first sign that the body is losing fat occurs when the clothes fit better. However, because loss of body fat is initially offset by increase in muscle tissue, there is normally little change in scale weight during the first several weeks. Once the increase in muscle tissue is complete, a process that takes approximately one month depending on body type, the second sign that the body is losing fat occurs when scale weight begins to decrease. At this point, it is just a matter of commitment and time for subjects to achieve their weight loss goals.

The Importance of Body Type

Depending on body type, the capacity to rebuild the body with power amino acids can take as little as one week (for those who have higher metabolic rates and higher activity levels) or as long as 1 month (for those who have lower metabolic rates and lower activity levels). Once a state of anabolic, supercharged health has been established with power amino acids, people begin to lose weight according to the table below:

Table 13-3

Body type	Metabolic Rates and Activity Levels	Time needed to begin rebuilding the body with power amino acids	Weight loss begins in
Type 1	Rapid metabolism Physically active	1 week	Week 2
Type 2	Rapid metabolism Physically inactive	2 weeks	Week 3
Type 3	Slow metabolism Physically active	3 weeks	Week 4
Type 4	Slow Metabolism Physically inactive	4 weeks	Week 5

In the beginning, subjects must show dedication, commitment, and patience. The rewards from persistence will be significant weight loss without intense exercise routines or strict dietary regimens and sustained weight control throughout life.

How to Accelerate Weight Loss with Power Amino Acids

Among the group of more than 700 patients who took the Factor4 regimen, we observed large variations in expectations and needs. Subjects varied greatly in the amount of weight they wanted to lose. They also varied in how fast they desired to lose excess weight. And finally, we assumed that their metabolic rates would vary according to age, gender, genetic profiles, and exercise levels.

Because of these variables in body weight and energy levels, we developed a weight management system with four steps or levels of increasing commitment to Factor4 shakes[1] and smoothies[2] to manage effective weight loss across a broad spectrum of individuals with different goals and requirements. As listed below, these levels are cumulative, meaning that higher levels of management include all lower levels of management as well.

Power level 1: Snack Control
The strategy at the first level of commitment is to take the Factor4 formula in lieu of snacks to block excess intake of carbohydrate-rich foods, including candy, chips, pastries, and ice cream. Factor4 works immediately to block food cravings, hunger pangs, famished states, and eating binges. The Factor4 formula should be taken at least twice daily in this program.

Power Level 2: Portion Control
The strategy at the second level of commitment includes taking Factor4 formula prior to or with meals to minimize food intake with portion control. Thus, Factor4 allows individuals to eat half meals and reduce the number of calories ingested throughout the day without suffering from hunger attacks. The Factor4 formula should be taken at least 2 to 3 times per day in this program.

Power Level 3: Meal Replacement
The strategy at the third level of commitment includes taking Factor4 as meal replacements once or twice daily to reduce the number of calories ingested throughout the day even further. Dinner may consist of a source

of protein (fish, chicken, or lean beef) and two vegetables (colored or leafy). The essential nutrients in Factor4 keep the body energized and satisfied with minimal consumption of food calories. Factor4 should be taken at least 3 to 4 times per day in this program.

Power Level 4: Boot Camp

The strategy at the fourth level of commitment includes taking Factor4 power shakes at 3 to 4 hour intervals throughout the day to maximize high-value nutrients that burn fat while minimizing low-value nutrients (carbohydrates and fat) that lead to fat deposition. Factor4 should be taken at least four to five times per day for women and men, respectively, in this program. Two modest-sized meals are allowed at this power level.

- One meal, allowed in the morning, may consist of fresh fruit, an orange, a half-grapefruit, plums, berries or melons. No sugar is allowed on the fruit.
- Another meal, allowed in the evening, may consist of vegetables that contain between 5% and 10% carbohydrate (salad greens, spinach, broccoli, asparagus, kale, cucumbers, pickles, onions or colored vegetables such as carrots, peppers, beets or okra). Eat as many of these vegetables as you like at a single sitting. Steam the vegetables and serve them sprayed with "I Can't Believe It's Not Butter — Spray." This spray, which is very tasty on steamed vegetables, contains minimal calories (<10) and less than 1 g of unsaturated fat. Minimal amounts of low-calorie dressing may be served on the side with salad greens.
- Crispy rye crackers are permitted as a high fiber source with minimal digestible carbohydrate.

The number of days per week that power level 4 is followed may vary depending on the needs of the individual and their weight-loss goals[3]. Many people follow this regimen for 48 hours (2 days) each week and move down to power level 3 for the remainder of the week. Others who are more aggressive in their weight loss goals follow power level 4 for longer periods of time, from 3 to 6 days per week and move down to power level 3 on the last day of the week. All participants are surprised at how good their bodies feel during "boot camp" at power level 4. Most marvel at the complete absence of hunger on fruits, vegetables and Factor4. That is the marvelous power of Factor4!

The Power Chain of Factor4 in Weight Control

Once excess weight loss has been achieved, it is possible for individuals to move down the power chain to a lower value. For example, if someone has selected power level 4 to lose 80 pounds of weight over a 6 month period, they may be able to move down the power chain to power level 3, then to power level 2, and finally to power level 1 to maintain sustained weight control.

Naturally, individuals who begin to gain excessive weight again can move up the power chain to levels 2, 3, or 4 to block further weight gain, reverse the trend in body weight shifts, and again achieve weight loss health.

The real secret of the Factor4 weight management program is that it contains the essential nutrients (power amino acids, protein, vitamins, and minerals) that are necessary to reset metabolic pathways so they optimize fat-burning metabolism in the body. It does this without resorting to starvation mechanisms that harm the body by compromising vital organs and muscle tissue that are necessary for optimal health.

Because individuals can move up and down the Factor4 power chain, replacing one power level strategy with another to offset unwanted shifts in body weight, the Factor4 regimen can be used by anyone to regulate body weight without causing the catabolic (destructive) effects of popular diets and weight loss gimmicks on metabolic health.

Exercise

Naturally, vigorous exercise will accelerate weight loss according to the intensity of workout routines. However, by following the Factor4 process, dieters do not need to engage in intense exercise routines or even strict dietary regimens. By correcting the deficiencies in amino acids, positive-charged proteins, and metabolic pathways, this program works naturally, through nature's own pathways, to stimulate weight loss and achieve sustained weight control.

However, exercise should be an important part of daily life for anyone who is interested in achieving optimal body fitness.

What Other Changes Need to Be Made in the Diet?

Much of this book has described in detail the harmful effects of refined sugars, high-density carbohydrates, saturated fats, and trans fats in the development of overweight disorders and obesity. It is necessary to reduce these harmful foods in the diet to achieve the full power of supercharged health with power amino acids. Many of the recommendations shown below have been recognized for years to be effective tools in weight management. Here are the additional changes that need to be made:

- Lower your intake of refined sugars (sucrose or high fructose corn syrup) by 90% or more
- Avoid soft drinks, colas, and energy drinks altogether
- Because of the sugars added to processed fruit juices, reduce these by at least 50% or replace them with the natural fruit itself
- Except on rare occasions, say NO to sugar-rich foods such as candy, cakes, pies, cookies, ice cream, pastries, and sticky buns
- If you add sugar, sugar substitutes, and/or cream or milk to coffee, consider switching to tea and taking it without any adulterants
- Cut high density, starch-rich carbohydrate foods by half. This means portion control, reducing portion sizes by at least 50% for bread, potatoes, white rice, flour, pasta, noodles, and pizza. Pass on the bread-basket in restaurants and at home
- By reducing starch-rich foods, you will make room for so-called "superfoods": vegetables, fruits, and nuts that are rich in fiber and phytonutrients (antioxidants). Eat as many of these brightly colored super-foods as possible. Variety is important, as the USDA recommends
- Minimize or avoid saturated fats, especially those in processed foods such as pies, cakes, butter, salad dressings, rich sauces, and ice cream. All fat-containing dressings, sauces, and butter should be ordered "on the side" and used with great care
- Avoid desserts loaded with sugar and saturated fat, including cakes, cookies, and pies at home or on the road. In restaurants or on special occasions, share a single dessert with multiple friends and enjoy the pleasures of taste without the dietary impact of excessive calories.

Once you have used the Factor4 regimen of power amino acids to lose your "sweet tooth," one or two spoonfuls of a rich dessert will be more than enough!

- At home, serve a wide variety of fruits and berries for dessert. Choose natural fruits that have limited amounts of sugar. Particularly tasteful are berries (strawberries, blueberries, blackberries, raspberries, and cranberries) covered with soymilk or low-fat milk
- Avoid table salt, salt-rich foods, and minimize the use of salt in cooking

The Carbohydrate Challenge

Earlier chapters in this book have focused on the role of refined sugars and high-density carbohydrates in obesity disorders and the diseases of civilization that lead to accelerated aging through the Metabolic Syndrome. Carbohydrate-rich diets lead to uncontrolled hunger and uncontrolled weight gain by encouraging high blood sugar, high blood insulin levels, and insulin resistance.

Much of the weight loss challenge has to do with managing carbohydrate intake. Refined sugars must be limited at all costs. Although complex carbohydrates are healthier than refined sugars, they deserve special discussion, since they show considerable variations in caloric content according to density.

- High density, starch-rich vegetables that contain 45–65% carbohydrates include bread, pasta, pizza, white rice, white flour, muffins, bagels, croissants, and cinnamon rolls
- Vegetables that contain 20% carbohydrates include potatoes (white, red, and yellow) and sweet potatoes
- Vegetables that contain 15% carbohydrates include green peas, green beans, and artichokes
- Vegetables that contain 10% carbohydrates include onions and colored vegetables, such as carrots, beets, and okra
- Vegetables that contain 5% carbohydrates are largely green vegetables, including lettuce, spinach, broccoli, asparagus, kale, cucumbers, and pickles

It is important to replace high-density, starch-rich foods with lower calorie vegetables as much as possible. Because of their caloric density, starch-rich foods can be harmful in attempts to balance the caloric equation.

The Fat Challenge

In order to achieve supercharged health, both high-density carbohydrate and saturated fat need to be restricted in the diet. However, it makes more sense to avoid the fat in processed foods than the fat in meat and chicken products. Man evolved over 2 million years eating high-protein, high-fat foods obtained from the natural environment. Metabolic pathways in humans can handle the fat that accompanies most fish, poultry, and meat products. The fats used in processed foods, however, have often been modified or transformed by hydrogenation into trans fats that are poorly metabolized in the human body.

The sensible way to meet the fat challenge is to follow the simple rules below:

- Select lean cuts of red meat, such as New York steak, tenderloin, filet mignon, and top and bottom round steaks. Remove all visible fat before cooking
- Broil, bake, or barbeque. Do not fry anything
- Steam vegetables and season them with herbs and spices instead of butter and sauces
- Sauté or poach fish, chicken, and other foods with wine or defatted broth. Use olive oil sparingly
- Use non-fat milk, 1% fat milk, or soy milk and non-fat or low-fat cheese
- Use low-fat salad dressings at home. In restaurants ask for salad dressings, rich sauces, and butter "on the side" and use them sparingly
- Avoid processed foods that are high in fat, including crackers, chips, cookies, cakes, pie and popcorn, and particularly avoid those made with hydrogenated oil (trans-fat), palm oil, or cocoa butter
- Purchase products in which mono- and poly-unsaturated fats have replaced saturated fats

Thus, even after weight loss has been achieved, dietary carbohydrate and fat, particularly saturated fat, need to be restricted. Not all fats are the same. It makes more sense to avoid the fat in processed foods than the fat in meat and chicken products. Metabolic pathways can handle the fat that accompanies most poultry and meat products when taken in moderation. The fats used in processed foods, however, have often been modified or transformed in ways that make them unrecognizable to human metabolic processes.

To understand the beneficial and harmful effects of different kinds of fats, it is instructive to review the spectrum of fats from healthy to unhealthy in the following table.

Table 13-4

Fat	Food source	Health status
Monounsaturates	Nuts, avocados, canola oil, olive oil	Lower LDL (bad) cholesterol raises HDL (good) cholesterol
Polyunsaturates	Corn and soy oils; fish, flaxseed, soybeans, tofu, walnuts, Heart healthy omega-3s	lower LDL (bad) cholesterol
Saturated fats	Meats, full-fat dairy, tropical oils	Raise LDL (bad) cholesterol lowers HDL (good) cholesterol
Trans fat in hydrogenated vegetable oils	Cookies, crackers, deep-fried foods	Appear to be even more harmful than saturated fat

Achieve Supercharged Health and Superior Weight Control with Power Amino Acids

We formulated Factor4 as a prototypical way of delivering power amino acids, protein, vitamins, minerals, and micronutrients to the human body. As shown in Chapter 10, the Factor4 regimen outperformed four popular diets in weight loss success. The four popular diets span the great divide in American diets over the past 60 years. The results speak for themselves. When monitored by unbiased observers, the four popular diets led to remarkably small reductions in weight. The average weight loss experienced after 6 months with the Factor4 regimen significantly exceeded the average weight loss experienced after 12 months with any of these diet plans. Over the course of a year, the Factor4 regimen showed weight-loss performance that was greater than 3 times more effective than the front-runner among the popular diets and greater than 5 times more effective than the other three diets (See Table 10-1).

Time-Honored Dietary Principles

In addition to reviewing the Factor4 breakthrough diet that will allow you to lose significant weight with a regimen of power amino acids, it is important to review some of the time-honored dietary principles that still apply in the quest to achieve better health. This section, which is focused on health food categories and healthy weight pyramids, is inspired by *The Mayo Clinic Plan: 10 Essential Steps to a Better Body and Healthier Life* and by the USDA website at www.mypyramid.com. Let us first consider the major food categories.

Vegetables and Fruits

Fresh produce in the form of vegetables and fruit is the first component of the food pyramid because it is the healthiest of the dietary staples. Vegetables and fruits are rich in essential vitamins, phytonutrients, and antioxidants, including beta carotene and vitamin C. They are key sources of essential minerals, including potassium and magnesium, which are important in the control of blood pressure. They are rich in fiber that may stabilize blood sugar, lower cholesterol levels, and increase regularity in intestinal function.

Studies show that people who regularly eat generous portions of fruits and vegetables show a lower risk for the leading causes of death in America, including cardiovascular disease, high blood pressure, diabetes, and cancer. Many fruits contain generous amounts of flavinoids, which work together to lower the risks of heart disease and cancer. Some fruits and vegetables contain the antioxidants, lutein and zeaxanthines, which may help guard against aging as well as against eye diseases, including macular degeneration. Some nuts are rich in beta-sistosterol, which is believed to help lower blood cholesterol.

Because of their many benefits, there are no limits to the daily servings of brightly-colored fresh and frozen vegetables and fruits. The exceptions are dried fruits and fruit juices that contain significantly higher levels of sugar than fresh fruit and therefore should be avoided or reduced in portion size.

The following table lists healthy fruits, vegetables and legumes.

Table 13-5

Fruits	Vegetables	Legumes*
Half banana	Carrots	White & navy beans
Half grapefruit	Green beans	Lima beans
1 cup of grapes	Broccoli	Pinto and black beans
1 cup of strawberries	Cauliflower	Black-eyed peas
1 cup of blueberries	Salad greens	Split peas
1 cup of backberries	Squash	Brown and red lentils
1 cup of cranberries	Spinach	Chick peas
Tomatoes		

* Legumes are vegetable sources that contain increased amounts of protein. Accordingly, they are also listed with protein and dairy.

The virtue in fruits and vegetables lies in their low energy density, which means a large portion contains only a few calories. For example, one vegetable serving contains only about 25 calories; one fruit serving contains only about 60 calories. Hence, the Mayo Clinic Plan recommends 4 or more vegetable servings per day and 3 or more fruit servings a day.

Carbohydrates

High-density or starch-rich carbohydrates are available either as whole grains, with minimal processing, or white grains, with extensive processing. Whole grains consist of the outer layers, known as the bran and germ, and the starch-rich interior, called the endosperm. During the processing of whole grains into white bread or white rice, the grains lose protein and many of their natural vitamins, phytonutrients, and most of their fiber. Potatoes are a good example. Potato skins are full of nutrients, including protein and fiber, while the white center consists of high-density starch.

It is wise to choose whole grain pastas, breads, and cereals and to serve brown rice rather than white rice. The less refined a carbohydrate food, the better it is for your health. Table 13-6 lists high-density carbohydrates that are considered healthy.

Notice that no sugars or sugar drinks are included in this table. The harmful effects of refined sugars have been discussed elsewhere in this book. Because high-density, starch-rich carbohydrates add abundant calories to diets, their portion sizes should be tightly controlled, as recommended earlier in this chapter.

Table 13-6

High Density Carbohydrates	
½ cup dry cereal	½ whole grain English muffin
1 slice whole grain bread	1 slice whole wheat bread
½ cup of cooked bulgur	½ cup cooked whole wheat pasta
½ large baked sweet potato	½ cup oatmeal
½ cup shredded wheat	½ whole-grain bagel

Protein and Dairy

It is not necessary or even desirable to eat meat everyday, especially if you are supplementing your diet with the Factor4 regimen of power amino acids described in this book. Many cuts of chicken, turkey, beef, lamb, and pork are high in saturated fat and cholesterol. Other foods that are rich sources of protein are low-fat dairy products, seafood, and many plant foods, including spinach and legumes. Legumes, including beans, lentils, and peas, are good sources of protein because they contain no cholesterol and little fat. They also make great complementary side dishes with meat or poultry.

In contrast to meat, beans help reduce LDL (bad) cholesterol levels, and the minerals they contain help to control blood pressure. Soybeans contain a complete set of nonessential and essential amino acids. The deficiencies in amino acids in other beans may be offset by a regimen of power amino acids as described in this chapter.

Fish and shellfish are excellent sources of protein and some represent rich sources of omega-3 fatty acids as well. Fish is low in calories, saturated fat, and cholesterol and therefore makes a good substitute for poultry and meat. Research suggests that most people would benefit by eating at least 2 servings of fish a week. Omega-3 fatty acids in fish (salmon, mackerel, and herring are rich sources) help lower triglycerides, the fat-rich particles in the bloodstream that appear to raise the risk of cardiovascular disease. They may also help prevent cardiac arrhythmias (dangerous heart beat disturbances) and help regulate blood pressure and improve immune function.

The following table lists healthy protein-containing foods, including fish, poultry, meat, eggs, dairy, and legumes.

Table 13-7

Fish, Poultry, Meat & Eggs	Dairy	Legumes
3 oz fish	1 cup of low-fat milk	1 cup of soy milk
3 oz chicken	1 cup of fat and sugar-free	Half cup of tofu
3 oz of turkey	yogurt	Half cup of cooked beans
2–3 oz lean beef	¼ cup of low-fat cottage,	Soy protein
2–3 oz of lamb	feta, ricotta or cream	
2–3 oz of pork	cheese	
2–3 oz of buffalo	20–30g of whey protein	
2 egg whites daily	20–30g of casein protein	
1 egg daily		

Because protein-rich foods may add abundant fat calories to diets, their portion sizes should be tightly controlled, as recommended earlier in this chapter. The superiority of power amino acids to protein-rich foods and protein shakes in maintaining normal body weight and protein health was discussed in Chapter 12.

Fats

It is preferable to replace saturated animal fats with liquid vegetable oils. For example, canola and olive oils are rich in unsaturated fats and preferable to solid shortenings (butter) or margarine. Because "fat follows protein" in many meats, seafood, and dairy products, it is recommended that you choose low-fat and lean versions of these foods. Saturated fats from animal sources raise LDL (bad) and lower HDL (good) cholesterol. Choose low-fat dairy products, and combine lean meats with at least 2 servings of vegetables.

Avoid fat-rich salad dressings, cooking oils, and butter. Because of their high calorie contents, vegetable oils, including olive oil, are best used in moderation. Nuts often contain protein, thiamin, niacin, folate, selenium, vitamin E, and healthy unsaturated oils.

Table 13-8 lists healthy fats.

Because fats are inherently rich in calories (1 gram contains 9 calories compared to 4 calories for protein and 4 calories for carbohydrate), their portion sizes should be tightly controlled, as recommended earlier in this chapter.

Table 13-8

Healthy Fats	
7 almonds	4 walnut or pecan halves
1½ tsp of peanut butter	1 tbs sunflower seeds
9 large olives	1 tsp canola or olive oil
2-4 tbs fat-free mayonnaise	10 unsalted, roasted peanuts (in shell)

Chocolate

Some chocolates are healthy in that they contain large quantities of fla-vinoids. These natural anti-oxidants, also found in tea, red wine, and some fruits and vegetables, help limit the negative effects of LDL (bad) choles-terol. The darker the chocolate, the higher the likelihood it contains flavi-noids. Accordingly, white chocolate contains no flavinoids. Cocoa beans, from which chocolate is derived, also contain cocoa butter and high levels of sugar, both of which add fat and sugar calories. For example, 1 oz of semisweet chocolate contains 135 calories.

Fiber

Fiber is the indigestible components of vegetables and whole grains. Fiber is either soluble or insoluble depending on its solubility in water.

Insoluble Fiber

Insoluble fiber—roughage—promotes healthy digestion and bowel function. Most common vegetables and whole grains contain significant amounts of insoluble fiber, which has the following benefits:

- Fiber can absorb up to 30 times its own weight in water. Acting like a sponge, it can create softer, larger stools that serve to increase regu-larity and reduce digestive problems, including constipation, hemor-rhoids, and diverticulitis.
- By slowing the digestive process, fiber helps lower cholesterol levels and may reduce the risks of heart disease and stroke. Fiber also slows the absorption of sugar from the intestinal tract, stabilizing sugar levels in the blood stream and reducing the risk of diabetes.

- Fiber helps stabilize body weight because foods high in fiber contain minimal calories that not only slow the digestive process but may decrease the calories absorbed into the body.

Soluble Fiber

Through its ability to create gelatinous environments around food particles, soluble fiber may help lower serum cholesterol. Foods that are high in soluble fiber are oats, barley, peas, beans, and citrus fruits. Soluble fiber may also be metabolized by bacteria in the GI tract, giving rise to short-chain fatty acids, which lower the pH of the bowel lumen, particularly in the colon. Lower pH in the colon stimulates the growth of beneficial bacteria that act as a rich source of essential amino acids (see Chapter 11). In addition, the short-chain fatty acids produced by these bacteria are distributed throughout the body, leading to improved metabolic health.

Fiber Sources in Food

Experts recommend that humans take in 20 to 30 grams or more of fiber per day. The following vegetables, legumes, fruits, and whole grains are rich sources of fiber.

Table 13-9

Source and Portion	Approx grams
Apple small	2.8
Banana medium	2.0
Beans (kidney) half cup	5.5
Beans (Lima) half cup	4.4
Bread (whole wheat) Slice	2.0
Broccoli ¾ cup	5.0
Carrots (raw) 4 sticks	1.7
Green beans half cup	2.1
Green peas (canned) half cup	3.0
Oat bran half cup	3.0
Orange small	3.0
Peach medium	2.0
Potato small	4.2
Rice (brown) half cup	5.5
Rye Crisp Cracker	6.0
Watermelon thick slice	2.8

General Dietary Advice

It is important to develop a positive attitude about what you want to accomplish. And it is equally important that you "stay the course." Here are five "dietary don'ts" that you need to remember:

- Don't starve yourself. Eat three meals a day. If you are hungry in between meals, drink a shake or smoothie made with power amino acids. If you are hungry when mealtime rolls around, select most foods from the base of the healthy weight pyramid, including vegetables and fruits. Eat slowly and savor the flavor of good food and conversation.
- Don't put yourself on a timeline. The effort to change life-long behavior is a gradual process and doesn't happen overnight.
- Don't let occasional setbacks weaken your commitment. Expect them and know you can overcome them.
- Don't try to be perfect. You can always learn from your mistakes. And remember, "'perfect' is the enemy of 'good'."
- Don't give up or give in. Persistence leads to success. A lifestyle commitment to power amino acids will restore core body health and optimal body weight.

Food Pyramids

For individuals who prefer to see information presented in a visual context, it is instructive to compare the food pyramid that we recommend during active efforts to lose weight to the food pyramid we recommend for maintaining healthy body weight once excess weight is lost.

Weight Loss Pyramid

Figure 13-1 represents a food pyramid designed for active weight loss efforts. It is rich in the fruits and vegetables that provide fullness while minimizing the delivery of calories. Not surprisingly, high-density or starch-rich carbohydrates and saturated fats are reduced in this pyramid by 50% or more. Refined sugars are absent from the pyramid, and starch-rich carbohydrates are reduced as well. Anabolic health is maintained with power amino acids, dairy products (low-fat milk or soy milk), with or without modest portions of protein-rich foods. Hunger is satisfied with

Figure 13-1

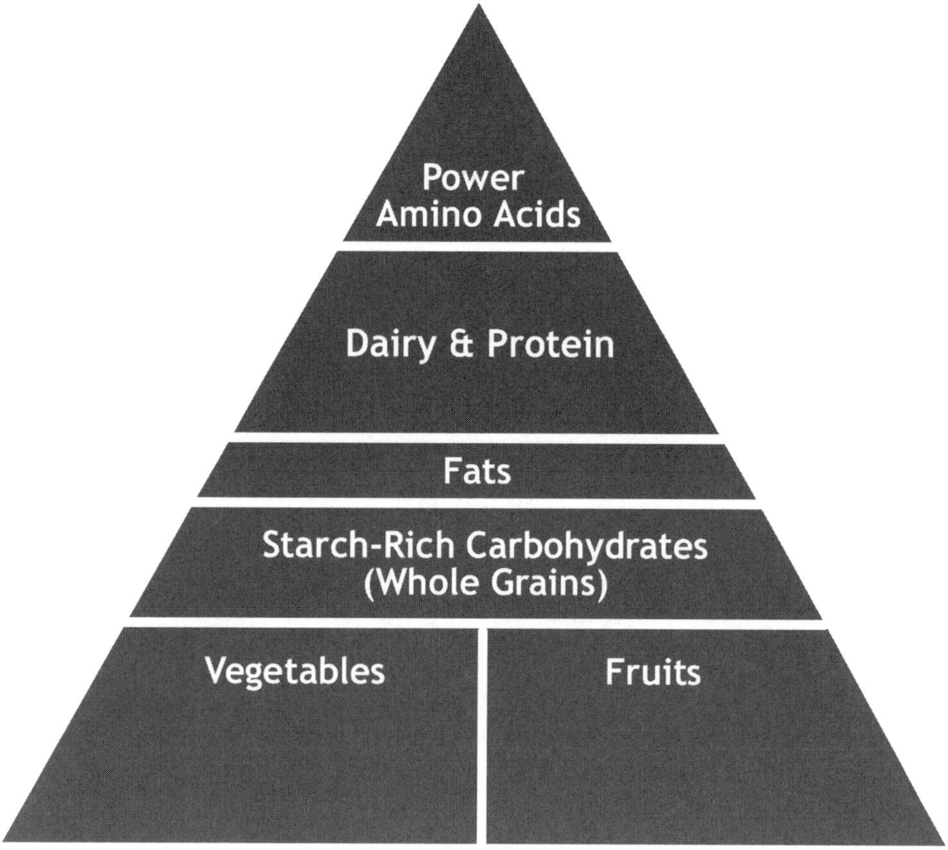

power amino acid shakes that confer feelings of comfort, satisfaction, and well-being as well as pep and energy.

The weight loss pyramid may be followed according to the four power levels in the weight management program described earlier in this chapter, which allows reductions in dietary calories roughly to 1,600 calories in power level 1, 1,400 calories in power level 2, 1,200 calories in power level 3, and 1,000 calories or less in power level 4. At the same time, anabolic health is maintained and appetite centers remain fully satisfied.

Weight Maintenance Pyramid

The food pyramid for sustained weight control is similar to that for active weight loss with one exception—calories return to normal levels. This pyramid continues to be rich in healthy vegetables and fruits. However, the limitations on high density carbohydrates and fat are reduced in accordance with energy expenditures, including exercise, that occur during the day. Refined sugars are still absent from the pyramid, and high density, starch-rich carbohydrates are still reduced by up to 25–50%. All reasonable efforts are made to minimize saturated fat and avoid trans-fats.

However, with the beneficial effects of power amino acids on metabolic pathways, the numbers of calories allowed by a maintenance pyramid rise to approximately 1,800 to 2,000 calories per day for women and approximately 2,400 to 2,800 calories per day for men. Naturally, the final set-points for calorie consumption depend on the weight of the individual, the amount of energy expended during the day, and the continued supplementation with power amino acids according to a maintenance regimen.

Summary

This chapter provides practical advice on using power amino acids in the form of power shakes and smoothies to treat deficiencies in amino acids, positive-charged proteins and metabolic pathways that cause the Metabolic Syndrome, which is associated with overweight disorders and other chronic degenerative diseases that lead to accelerated aging, enhanced suffering and early death. The chapter also explains what other changes need to be made in the diet to limit refined sugars, complex carbohydrates and saturated or hydrogenated fats.

Once supercharged health has been achieved with rebalanced amino acids, protein health and metabolic pathways, according to the general theory of nutrition reported in this book, it now becomes relatively easy to lose weight, regain metabolic health, revitalize youth and achieve anti-aging health, the four cornerstones of improved health and quality of life.

The dietary changes recommended in this Chapter for limiting the intake of dietary carbohydrate, including refined sugars, and increasing anabolic health with power amino acids, combine to provide four power levels of a low fat/carb diet that may be adjusted to the individual needs of patients for losing varying amounts of excess weight without resorting to catabolic diets that lead to extreme hunger. This approach allows us to avoid the limitations of both the high fat/protein diets promoted by Dr. Atkins and other physicians (rebound obesity as carbohydrate intake increases) and the low fat/protein diets promoted by public health policy (starvation hunger that leads to rebound obesity). The result is a revolutionary break-through in control of body weight as well as the Metabolic Syndrome that is associated with the chronic degenerative diseases that lead to accelerated aging and early death.

This chapter also reviews time-honored principles in dietary health and shows how these principles, expressed in healthy food choices, may be maintained during efforts to balance metabolic pathways that lead to body weight health. Finally, this chapter brings together all of the recommendations made throughout this book into a food pyramid that shows schematically the dietary strategies for using power amino acid regimens to achieve significant weight loss followed by sustained weight control.

The final chapter of the book will discuss the potential for supercharged health to combat nutritional and metabolic disease around the world in both advanced societies and underdeveloped nations.

Chapter 14

Metabolic Health, Aging and Human Dignity

The Toll of Poor Health in Today's World

According to the World Health Organization, more than one billion adults worldwide are overweight, and 300 million are obese. Obesity and related disorders are connected to four of the top 10 diseases identified throughout the world by the World Health Organization. These include obesity, high blood pressure, myocardial infarction and stroke, and cancer. Given these demographics, metabolic disease involves global suffering on a grand scale.

The Importance of Power Amino Acids and Supercharged Health in the Prevention and Treatment of Metabolic Diseases

Poor Protein Health

This book focuses on the importance of power amino acids—the 9 essential amino acids plus Arginine—in closing the food chain gap and achieving protein health. Optimal protein health means balanced protein health with full expression of positive-charged proteins as well as negative-charged proteins. By supplementing the diet with power amino acids, they act rapidly to correct deficiencies in essential amino acids, positive-charged proteins and metabolic pathways that lead to poor metabolic health and overweight disorders.

Overweight Disorders and Obesity

This book has defined "selective protein deficiency syndrome" as a deficiency in positive-charged proteins that may lead to metabolic defects, including overweight disorders and obesity. Because power amino acids close the gap in the food chain and re-establish protein health and metabolic pathways more rapidly than other nutritional strategies, these essential nutrients lead to rapid weight loss through power nutrition and supercharged health, appetite suppression, increased energy, and changes in metabolic pathways that result in loss of body fat.

Metabolic Syndrome and Accelerated Aging

It now appears that metabolic disorders and risk factors associated with Metabolic Syndrome may be responsible for accelerated aging and early death in increasing numbers of individuals. It appears that the Metabolic Syndrome is caused, in part, by dietary excess of simple sugars and complex carbohydrates that lead to multiple dysfunctions in carbohydrate metabolism, including hyperglycemia, hyperinsulinism, insulin resistance, protein glycation, formation of advanced glycation end products, and inflammatory reactions.

These abnormalities in carbohydrate metabolism result in a continuum of metabolic disorders, including obesity, type II diabetes, cardiovascular disease (heart attack, stroke, and peripheral vascular disease), hypertension, cancer, and a number of blood abnormalities associated with this spectrum of metabolic diseases, accelerated aging, and early death.

Power amino acids rapidly restore protein health, which helps curb the abnormalities in carbohydrate and fat metabolism that lead to the multiplicity of metabolic diseases described earlier as "diseases of civilization" and more recently as Metabolic Syndrome. By treating these metabolic abnormalities and risk factors, power amino acids appear to revitalize youth and may increase anti-aging health and longevity with improved quality of life.

Nutritional Disease in the Underdeveloped World

Because power amino acids restore protein health rapidly, they may be particularly useful in poorly nourished societies in the underdeveloped world. The metabolic priming and catabolic-releasing factors that accompany the use of power amino acids may result in the rapid relief of the nutritional deficiencies caused by protein starvation and the restoration of nutritional health to individuals who live in undernourished cultures.

The Importance of Protein and Metabolic Health in Quality of Life

Comfort, Satisfaction, and Well-being

Protein health is critical in dietary sustenance because it supports the metabolic health that optimizes quality of life. The central role of power amino acids in establishing protein health makes them fundamental to human health. Without protein health that leads to comfort, satisfaction, and well-being, we are left with metabolic abnormalities that compromise the enjoyment of life and adversely affect personal productivity, self-esteem, and human dignity.

A recent article in the *New York Times* documented increased "sugar swings" in the workplace due to soft drinks and power bars, both of which contain excesses of refined sugars and chemical sweeteners. "Food swings" frequently lead to "mood swings." Hunger frequently morphs into anger, giving rise to a new word, "hangry," a combination of "hungry" and "angry," and a new expression, "to be hangry." Furthermore, "I'm hungry" has become a culturally accepted rationalization for brusque behavior in the work place. One woman felt at ease to say, "I'm really hungry right now and I'm really sorry. Just give me half an hour and I'll be fine." Apparently, the "half hour" was needed to ingest a power bar!

Fortunately, power amino acids curb these food swings, rebalance metabolic pathways, and lead to comfort, satisfaction, and a sense of well-being.

Increased Pep and Energy

The pep, energy, activity, stamina, and endurance that come from power amino acids open the door to revitalized youth, something that almost every aging person seeks. These traits indicate that significant changes have occurred in the metabolic pathways of the body that lead to increased muscle tissue and decreased fat tissue.

Increased Quality of Life during the Aging Process

The aging process starts roughly at age 30 when hormone levels begin to decline in the human body. Aging begins slowly. It is not until their 40s, for example, that individuals with normal eyesight begin to need reading glasses. In their early 50s, women undergo menopause and men begin andropause. Joints may deteriorate, leading to arthritic pains. Posture may weaken. Sensory functions, like seeing and hearing, may wane. Taste and smell may become attenuated. Muscular strength decreases. Confidence wanes. Functions in each of the eight major health systems of the body begin to disappear. Body weight increases despite exercise and diets. The process of aging in today's world is not pretty.

However, the experience with power amino acid supplementation indicates that many of the characteristics of the aging process are due to nutritional factors related to "selective protein deficiency syndrome." By closing the food chain gap more efficiently with essential and positive-charged amino acids and avoiding the metabolic abnormalities of high carbohydrate diets, it may be possible to revitalize youth and significantly improve anti-aging health. Models of health and aging may be used to describe the potential benefits of power amino acids to society.

Figure 14-1A shows, in schematic fashion, the current relationships between health and age during the aging process. Beyond the age of thirty, most individuals experience a slow decline in metabolic health, which continues for the duration of life until a fatal illness occurs, as depicted in this diagram at age 70. Between age 30 and 68, there appears to be a significant decline in health, with a deterioration in quality of life due to the aging process.

However, many of these aging processes seem to be related to nutritional factors, particularly protein deficiency and carbohydrate excess. Since nutritional deficiencies appear to play a central role in the aging process, including the onset of chronic degenerative diseases, it may be possible to reverse these physical disorders and restore balanced protein health with power amino acids. Ultimately, it may be possible to develop a model of aging in which physical health does not steadily decline until death.

Figure 14-1B shows another model of aging health in which the natural course of aging sets in over the age of 30 and physical health declines until the age of 50. In this particular model, the subject begins to re-establish metabolic health at age 50 by taking dietary supplements of power amino acids, which lead, through feedback mechanisms, to a reduction in dietary carbohydrates. These subjects may be expected to halt the aging process and achieve a new plateau of improved health without further deterioration. It is also possible that some individuals will reverse the aging process and regain the plateau of health they experienced at maturity. As shown in Figure 14-1B, the plateau of health continues until the subject contracts a fatal illness in older age, depicted here at age 85.

A third model of aging health may also be considered. In Figure 14-1C, the subject begins taking supplements of power amino acids at age 30 and maintains power nutrition and supercharged health during the aging process. According to the assumptions of this model, the subject not only avoids many of the signs of aging but also may retain youthful health for a significantly longer period of time. Because power amino acids appear to combat the risk factors associated with the Metabolic Syndrome, it is conceivable that the subject may remain in good health for a longer period of time before a fatal illness intervenes. This would be consistent with the

Figure 14-1A

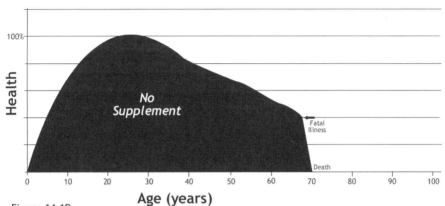

Figure 14-1B

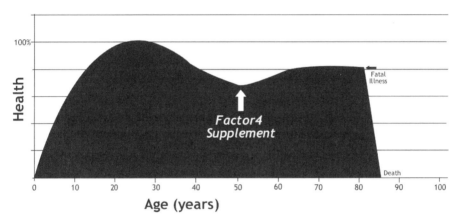

Figure 14-1C

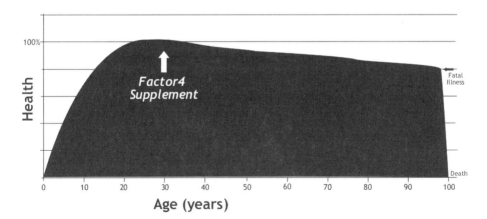

thesis that metabolic defects hasten the onset of lethal diseases or out-comes. In Figure 14-1C, the plateau of health is maintained almost until age 100.

Whichever model applies, the power amino acids that restore supercharged health with balanced protein expression may be expected to add years if not decades of anabolic health and revitalized youth to individual subjects.

The Importance of Metabolic Health in Personal Productivity

There are many reasons why personal productivity is compromised in our current society. This book has focused on the nutritional causes of Metabolic Syndrome, which appears to be the emerging cause of acceler-ated aging and early death around the world, not only in advanced cultures, but also in underdeveloped cultures as well.

The simple introduction of measures to improve protein health may be expected to both delay and combat the Metabolic Syndrome and lead to revitalized youth, anti-aging health, and increased longevity. The role of power amino acids in restoring protein health and avoiding carbohydrate overload in the eight major health systems in the body, including cardio-vascular health and aging health, may be expected to increase personal productivity on a grand scale.

Dependency Disorders and Drug Addictions

In addition to poor metabolic health and chronic degenerative diseases, dependency disorders, and drug addictions appear to increasingly augment the loss of personal productivity in both the advanced and underdeveloped worlds. An ever-expanding number of substances, including adulterated foods, alcohol products, and recreational drugs, play pivotal roles in the addictive disorders that are present in today's global society. However, many of these disorders may be beneficially managed with power amino acid supplementation, as described below.

Food Addictions
In the advanced world, food addictions have increased to epidemic pro-portions. Food addiction groups in the United States alone have increased 15-fold since the year 2000. This book has more than demonstrated the

serious consequences of metabolic disorders, including the Metabolic Syndrome, on overweight conditions and obesity as well as on chronic degenerative diseases, accelerated aging, and loss of personal productivity. At the same time, this book has demonstrated that power amino acids provide the most efficient means to correct the deficiencies in amino acids, positive-charged proteins, and metabolic pathways that lead to overweight disorders and obesity in the first place.

Alcohol Dependence and Addictions

Alcohol consumption is pervasive throughout society. Although moderate amounts of alcohol are believed to be harmless and even beneficial in some cases, chronic, excessive consumption of alcohol causes serious disease in most of the organs of the body, including the pancreas, liver, central nervous system, and muscles. The physical appearance of chronic alcoholics suggests grave nutritional defects. Muscle mass is wasted in the extreme, particularly in the arms and legs. Abdominal paunches (potbellies) appear in both alcoholic men and women. These effects indicate advanced catabolic states in alcoholic patients with concomitant losses in muscle tissues.

Prior to the onset of chronic alcoholism, alcoholic binging leads to considerable loss in productivity due to alcohol withdrawal (hangovers) and the metabolic consequences of excessive daily alcohol consumption. Alcohol is loaded with empty carbohydrate calories (6 calories per gram of alcohol), and beer is even more fattening, as it contains high levels of maltose sugars in addition to alcohol. Chronic alcoholism leads rapidly to protein deficiency disorders. Indeed, the increasing consumption of alcoholic beverages in America has contributed importantly to selective protein deficiency syndrome.

Not surprisingly, power amino acid supplements appear to treat alcohol-related disorders. In fact, power amino acids consumed before drinking alcohol decrease the rate of alcohol absorption and provide high-quality nutrients that may increase the metabolism of alcohol by the body. Power amino acids may also reduce the actual desire for alcohol and therefore decrease the amounts of alcohol consumed.

Taken during the recovery phase of alcoholic binge drinking, power amino acids confer additional benefits in re-establishing nutritional health. Preliminary studies have shown that the Factor4 regimen of amino acids restores fluid and mineral balance, provides nutritional support for the cardiovascular system, reducing tachycardias and arrhythmias, calms the digestive tract, and resets neurotransmitter profiles in the brain, helping to balance mood, combat depression, and promote restful sleep.

Power amino acids appear not only to treat the metabolic effects of alcohol but also to mitigate the addictive qualities of alcohol consumption. Their beneficial effects on neurotransmitter profiles, metabolic balance, nutritional health, and well-being may provide the relief necessary for alcoholics to reduce alcohol toxicity, reduce consumption, or possibly stop drinking altogether.

Drug Addictions

An increasing number of substances—including cocaine, heroin, crack, methamphetamines, pain killers, and steroids—feed drug-addiction disorders around the world. Most of these substances lead to addiction by altering neurotransmitter levels, not only in brain tissue but also throughout the body. Once these altered levels are established, the abrupt cessation of the substance leads to withdrawal symptoms that result from severe deficiencies in neurotransmitter profiles. The severity of withdrawal symptoms "chains" the subject to continued use of the substance. Addictive dependencies are unhealthy, demeaning, and frequently economically unsustainable.

Power amino acids appear to restore the levels of neurotransmitters throughout the body. This leads to enhanced feelings of comfort, satisfaction, and well-being that may prove beneficial for relieving the compulsions of addiction disorders.

The beneficial effects of power amino acids on neurotransmitter profiles, metabolic balance, nutritional health, and well-being may provide a powerful weapon in the war against dependency disorders and addictions that wreak havoc in the personal productivity of individuals who suffer from the debilitating effects of drugs. By effectively treating such disorders, power amino acids may be expected to increase significantly the productivity of such individuals in societies around the world.

The Importance of Metabolic Health in
Self Esteem and Human Dignity

It is well recognized that increased productivity leads to feelings of personal accomplishment. Especially for the young members of our society, improved metabolic health may well increase educational achievements in primary schools, high schools, colleges, and graduate schools. Higher educational levels may also produce more productivity that foster personal accomplishment and self-esteem.

For adults, improved metabolic health may not only increase personal productivity; it may also lead to more cohesive families who demonstrate greater love, satisfaction, and self-esteem.

For seniors, improved metabolic health may truly revolutionize the human life cycle. Currently seniors are relegated to retirement, overmedicated with poorly-indicated drugs, and eventually placed in nursing homes, where they are often forgotten altogether. Imagine if aging health could be improved to the point that senior members remain productive members of a cohesive, productive, and loving society. There would be no sense in keeping these seniors engaged in the highly competitive business ventures that are managed by younger adults. However, as these business ventures become more competitive and time-consuming, there will be an emerging need for healthy, productive seniors to play essential roles in the life cycle of human beings.

Thus, a revolutionary "Third Life" could be forged that would allow healthy seniors to fill critical roles in child-rearing, education, and community service, as well as creative roles in providing critical assistance to extended families. With increased flexibility in their schedules that allows for greater appreciation of life, senior citizens could continue to fulfill important roles in life and receive appropriate compensation for doing so.

Better health would lead to greater productivity. Continued financial compensation would lead to greater self-esteem and fulfillment in life. In short, the challenges of failing health that are now so prevalent in retirement communities could be replaced by a healthy, meaningful "Third Life" that benefits society as well as the senior citizens themselves. With improved metabolic health, revitalized youth, and increased longevity, senior citizens would have a real chance to enjoy personal significance and human dignity.

Dignity is defined in Webster's dictionary as "elevation of character," "intrinsic worth," and "achievement of excellence." By revitalizing youth and increasing longevity with improved quality of life, power amino acids could open the door to a new phase in the human life cycle: a "Third-Life" with increased wisdom, joy, and human dignity. This "Third-Life" might one day be recognized as the highest and most important phase of human existence.

The World Potential in Supercharged Health

Now imagine the benefits of supercharged health spread throughout the world. With relief from suffering in the four cornerstones of health, including body weight (both overweight and underweight), metabolic health, revitalized youth, and increased longevity with improved quality of life, productivity worldwide may be increased on an exponential scale.

Considerable progress could be achieved in treating both starvation and poor nutrition around the world. With improvements in protein health leading to supercharged health, young, adult, and senior citizens may all achieve significant increases in productivity, leading to greater fulfillment in family and professional activities.

With healthier parents and grandparents, extended families could function in more productive and cohesive ways. The greater spread in healthy ages could serve complementary purposes in the cycle of life. Senior citizens could become more involved in childcare, education, and community service, functions that are unfortunately lacking in today's world.

And the majority of disabilities caused by "diseases of civilization" and the Metabolic Syndrome may be greatly reduced, leading to enormous reductions in the cost of these disabilities to governments and societies alike. With increases in human productivity and decreases in health and entitlement costs, governments will be able to function more efficiently without having to add the growing burden of increased numbers of citizens who are dependent on government support programs.

In conclusion, the achievement of supercharged health around the globe may well increase the potential for establishing harmony among nations and sustaining life on this planet for years to come.

Notes

Chapter 1: The Great Divide in American Diets

1. Rudolph Schoenheimer started his career studying cholesterol metabolism in Germany but moved to New York City during World War II. While at Columbia University he developed the first biochemical assay for measuring cholesterol in the blood circulation.
2. In relationship to the later focus on protein health in this book, it is interesting to note that both diets recommend borderline low protein levels.
3. In this study 362,000 middle-aged men were followed and screened. The age-adjusted 6-year death rate per 1,000 men was plotted against serum cholesterol (mg/dl). This study concluded that the association between cholesterol and heart disease applied to any level of serum cholesterol.
4. The body mass index (BMI) is defined as the ratio between body weight and height (body weight in kilograms divided by height in meters squared). Metabolic states related to body weight have been defined according to BMI as shown in the table below:

BMI	Classification
>30	Obesity
25 – 30	Overweight
18.5 – 25	Normal
<18.5	Underweight
<17.5	Anorexia Nervosa
15	Starvation

Those with a BMI between 18.5 and 25 are considered normal in body weight. Adults with a body mass index between 25 and 30 are considered overweight. Adults with a BMI of 30 or more are considered obese. Those with a BMI of 35 or more may be considered morbidly obese. At the upper end of the scale this equation works for almost everyone except weight lifters. At the lower end of the scale, the World Health Organization considers anyone with a BMI below 18.5

as underweight; a BMI below 17.5 is one of the criteria for anorexia nervosa; a BMI near 15 is usually used as an indicator for starvation.

5. The states with the highest percentage of obesity are Mississippi, Alabama, West Virginia, Louisiana, and Tennessee. The states with the lowest percentage of obesity are Colorado, Massachusetts, Rhode Island, Connecticut, Vermont, and Montana. The federal government has set a goal of a 15% obesity rate by the year 2010. As of 2008, no state has met that goal.

6. Margaret Ohlson picked up where Pennington stopped and designed her own version of Pennington's diet, restricting both carbohydrates and calories. It was based on consuming 1,400 to 1,500 calories a day composed of 24% protein, 54% fat and 22% carbohydrate. In 16-week tests on seven women with mild to overt obesity, subjects lost between 19 and 37 pounds. "Without exception, the low-carbohydrate reducing diet resulted in satisfactory weight losses," Ohlson wrote. 'The subjects reported feelings of well-being and satisfaction. Hunger between meals was not a problem." One hundred fifty women put on diverse diets over the next 10 years found the low-fat diets "dry, uninteresting and hard to eat." On the other hand, her subjects found high-fat diets with 700 to 800 calories of fat to be much more satisfying.

7. Charlotte Young followed in Ohlson's footsteps. In her study of 16 overweight women and 8 overweight males on a 1,800-calorie high fat/protein diet, subjects lost between 9 and 28 pounds, averaging between 2 and 3 pounds per week. They were "unanimous in saying that they had not been hungry." The unfortunate but perhaps predictable result, in the words of Gary Taubes, was that "Ohlson's and Young's journal articles were ignored."

Chapter 2: Diseases of Civilization

1. *Physiological and Medical Observations among the Indians of Southern United States and Northern Mexico.*

Chapter 3: Adaptation of the Body to Changing Diets

1. Dr. Patrick O'Farrell developed a similar procedure for the separation of bacterial proteins at about the same time.

2. Co-authors who participated in scientific investigations that used the 2-dimensional gel electrophoresis procedure for basic research and dietary studies include researchers from two laboratories. Researchers in my laboratory at the Rockefeller University included George Palade, Alan Tartakoff, Diana Bartelt, Jessica Pash, Russell Jacoby, Gerhard Rohr and Wilfried Bieger. Colleagues in our sister laboratory at the Philipps University in Marburg, Germany, included Horst Kern, Jurgen Schick, Uli Rausch, Henrich Lutcke, Panayiotis Vasiloudes, Klaus Rudiger, Rita Verspohl, H. Beil-Moeller and Anna Fakadej.

Chapter 4: Energy Pathways within the Body

1. Metabolism in the body is carried out via metabolic pathways. In order to build (synthesize) protein, fat, and carbohydrate molecules in the body or breakdown (digest, degrade, and hydrolyze) these same molecules, these synthetic and hydrolytic processes are carried out through metabolic pathways.

   These pathways may be thought of as molecular assembly lines that assemble (build) and disassemble (breakdown) all the molecules that are important for cellular function. They are analogous to assembly lines in automobile manufacturing facilities. Each worker in the assembly line has a specific function to perform in the assembly of an automobile or truck. In metabolic pathways, the "workers" are called "enzymes," and each enzyme performs a specific function in the assembly or disassembly of molecules.

   Any given cell has thousands of enzymes that are organized in synthetic and hydrolytic—or metabolic—pathways to build and breakdown protein, fat, and carbohydrate molecules so that the cell can use them to carry out all of its cellular functions. Many of these proteins, fats, and carbohydrates act as the "bricks and mortar" that give rise to the basic structure of the cell. Other proteins, fats, and carbohydrates may exist in storage compartments (muscle, adipose tissue, and liver glycogen) from which they can be called forth for energy purposes in the body.

   For example, the Krebs cycle that exists in the mitochondria of all cells contains the metabolic pathways that complete the breakdown of proteins, fat, and carbohydrates and convert the energy of their chemical bonds into short-term energy reserves (ATP) that fulfill the energy requirements of the thousands of enzymes that drive all of the metabolic pathways in the cell.

The sum total of metabolic pathways include the thousands of metabolic processes in the cell. Together, the multiplicity of these processes and pathways may be called metabolism.

2. Mitochondria are intracellular organelles (compartments), vestiges of early bacteria, that act as cellular generators to produce energy as adenosine tri-phosphate (ATP) for body metabolism. Mitochondria use a combination of molecular pumps, carriers, electron transport proteins, and enzymes to convert energy extracted from the chemical bonds of dietary nutrients into ATP, which is then used to energize the enzymes that drive the numerous metabolic pathways within the cell.

3. Homeostasis is the process by which the organism maintains equilibrium, or balance, with respect to the various functions of the body that are related to chemical compositions of the molecules, cells, tissues, and fluids of the body. Some examples of these functions are temperature, heart rate, blood pressure, water content, blood sugar, and energy (ATP) levels.

In the course of evolution, organisms have acquired a remarkable collection of regulatory mechanisms for maintaining homeostasis at the molecular, cellular, and organism levels. When the steady state is disturbed by some change in external circumstances or energy supply, the temporarily altered fluxes through individual metabolic pathways trigger regulatory mechanisms intrinsic to each pathway. The net effect of all these molecular and energy adjustments is to return the organism to a new steady state that protects the current health status of the organism—that is to achieve homeostasis.

Chapter 5: Hormones Regulate Energy Pathways and Appetite

1. As discussed in this chapter the appetite center (ARC nucleus) contains two distinct neural networks, one with anorexigenic activity (appetite suppression) and one with orexigenic activity (appetite stimulation). 5 Hydroxy Tryptophan (5-HT) and its metabolite, serotonin, both stim-

ulate POMC neurons which are anorexigenic and inhibit agRP neuronal activity which are orexigenic. Both of these effects reinforce one another and lead to a reduction in food intake. Neuroanatomical, electrophysiological, transgenic and behavioral studies summarized most recently in Heisler, L.K., et al. 2006. Neuron, 51: 239-249 indicate that the central melanocortin system in the ARC nucleus is the key site of action of both 5-HT and Serotonin in the stimulation of hypophagia.

In the mid 1990s, Phen-Fen (Phentermine & Fenfluramine) was marketed for overweight disorders and obesity. This drug combination increased the level of serotonin, which suppressed appetite and shut down the action of dopamine on the "food reward pathway." As a result of its anorexigenic activity the sense of urgency to pursue food disappeared. Patients who felt hungry "all the time" lost much of their interest in food. In the grocery store they bought less food and their interest in junk food was reduced. Many of these patients claimed for the first time they "felt normal." Unfortunately, Phen-Fen had side effects which caused heart valve dysfunction and was pulled from the market in 1997.

Chapter 6: Fat Distribution in the Body

1. Previous studies have focused on one member of this family, Sirt1, which is activated by high doses of resveratrol, a substance found in red grapes, which has been shown, at very high concentrations approaching 1,000 fold levels observed in red wine, to prevent diabetes from developing and also prolong life in mice. This finding has generated tremendous attention in the commercial world, leading biotechnology and pharmaceutical companies to begin developing drugs and supplements to harness this effect.

2. Recent studies at the Joslin Diabetic Clinic at Harvard Medical School in Boston by Yu-Hua Tseng's team examined the factors that determine the amounts of different types of fat cells in the body. They identified a protein called BMP7 that promotes the creation of brown fat. Without this protein, the brown fat in mice was marginally low.

Chapter 7: Sugar: Pure, Sweet, and Deadly

1. While the glycemic index response to specific foods was reasonably consistent, different individuals showed varying responses, and the variations from day-to-day were "tremendous," as Wolever stated.

Chapter 8: The Metabolic Syndrome, Obesity, and Accelerated Aging

1. Toll-like receptors (TLR) have recently been implicated in the metabolic consequences of obesity, often termed metabolic syndrome, which is accompanied by lipotoxicity, inflammation and insulin resistance and leads to type 2 diabetes, atherosclerosis, hypertension and cardiovascular disease. Lipotoxicity is thought to result from overloading the body's ability to handle dietary lipids, especially saturated fatty acids. In humans TLR4 expression is up-regulated in muscle or adipose tissue from obese or type 2 diabetes patients and this increase correlates with insulin resistance and TLR4-mediated NFkB activation.

   Treatment of isolated muscle with saturated fatty acids (palmitate) activates signal transduction pathways (JNK and IKK/ NFkB), which also promote insulin resistance and enhances cellular output of inflammatory cytokines such as IL-6 and TNF-alpha. Interestingly, monounsaturated-fatty acids such as olein, which is enriched in olive oil, appear to neutralize the effects of palmitate. Exercise also has a positive effect, down-regulating the expression of TLR4 and decreasing fat accumulation in human muscle.

   Toll-like receptors were first discovered in relationship to the innate immune system, where they recognize bacterial lipopolysaccharides. At high concentrations, dietary lipids can also be recognized by TLR4 and to a lesser extent, TLR2, which activate the immune system in response to a diet rich in long-chain saturated fatty acids. Recent transgenic mice studies with loss-of-function mutation in the TLR4 receptor showed resistance to becoming obese on a high fat diet. Consequently, toll-like receptors appear to link many of the metabolic consequences of obesity due to high dietary intake of saturated fat..

Chapter 9: The Paradoxes of Nutritional Disease and Obesity in an Advanced Society

1. Powerbars are loaded with glycerol, which is one of the precursors to fat.

Chapter 10: Selective Protein Deficiency Syndrome and Obesity

1. Protein expression means two things. First, it means that the protein is produced by the organ or tissue. In this meaning the words "produced", "synthesized" and "expressed" are synonymous. Second, it can also relate to the amount of expression or the amount of protein that is synthesized or produced by the organ or tissue.

2. Selective protein deficiency syndrome is presented as a new entity that describes the continuum that exists in protein deficiency disorders between normal function and Kwashiorkor, which represents a far-advanced form of protein deficiency that presages accelerated aging and early death in underdeveloped countries. Early forms of Selective Protein Deficiency Syndrome (SPDS) in the advanced world are believed to be characterized by reduced expression of positive-charged proteins as depicted in Figures 10-1A, 10-1B and 10-1C. SPDS should not be confused with Kwashiorkor that can be expected to dramatically reduce the expression of both negative- and positive-charged proteins.

   Just as Metabolic Syndrome represents a continuum of metabolic disorders between normal, Metabolic Syndrome and Type 2 diabetes and/or cardiovascular disease, SPDS represents a continuum of protein deficiency disorders that define a pathway from normal to Selective Protein Deficiency Syndrome to Kwashiorkor.

   As such SPDS represents intermediate states of protein deficiency between normal expression of enzymes and metabolic pathways to far advanced states of SPDS represented by severe dysfunctions in Kwashiorkor, as reviewed in citations 41 and 66 in Appendix II, Publications by George A. Scheele, M.D., on Pancreatic Function.

   Metabolic pathways depend on amino acid and protein health. When the body suffers from "Selective Protein Deficiency Syndrome" due to an imbalance in essential and nonessential amino acids, positive-charged amino acids and proteins disappear long before negative-charged amino acids and proteins disappear. When there is an imbalance between the positive- and negative-charged proteins that serve as enzymes, the metabolic pathways become partially impaired as well, and this leads to poor health and accelerated aging.

Hence, power amino acids are critical for correcting the deficiencies in amino acids, proteins, and metabolic pathways so that the cells in the body can return to maximal or supercharged health.

Once we understand the role of diet in maintaining the complete set of amino acids, proteins, and metabolic pathways in the body, it becomes possible to understand why poor dietary habits and poor digestive functions during the aging process lead to imbalances in amino acids, proteins, and metabolic pathways that result in compromised health and aging.

Given that administering power amino acids to suffering human subjects produces improved metabolic health, weight loss, and revitalized youth, the cause and effect postulates appear to be initially established for the beneficial effects of power amino acids in human nutrition, metabolic health, body weight, and anti-aging effects as well.

3. The two negative-charged amino acids, aspartic acid and glutamic acid, are produced by the human body.

4. All patients in the weight loss study were monitored weekly according to body weight, body fat, lean body weight, body mass index (BMI) and body water by a certified personal trainer. All patients who lost weight showed significant decreases in their BMI. The entire study was closely monitored by a board certified physician in internal medicine. The design of the study and individual weight-loss curves may be viewed on www.factor4health.com.

Chapter 11: General Theory of Nutrition and Weight Control

1. It should be acknowledged here that both nonessential and essential amino acids are necessary for complete protein health. Accordingly, we do not make the claim that humans or other mammals can exist on supplementation with essential or "power" amino acids alone. To ensure that both nonessential and essential amino acids are readily available in the Factor4 weight loss diet, we include, in addition to the "power amino acid com-

plex," at least 10 grams of purified protein. The rationale for including both ingredients in the Factor4 regimen is discussed in Chapter 13.

2. Branched chain amino acids are popular in health food stores and among body builders and people who exercise.

3. These four factors provide an additional reason for referring to the regimen of power amino acids as "Factor4 health."

4. In the 2004 edition of their textbook, *Cell Biology,* Thomas Pollard and William Earnshaw cite the following (page 372):

> "The process of formation and degradation of autophagic vacuoles in the liver requires less than 15 minutes. Because large volumes of cytoplasm and entire organelles are destroyed, macroautophagy must be regulated precisely and directly. Although the exact nature of the intracellular messenger that triggers this highly choreographed process is unknown, the signal is thought to be tied to the intracellular levels of particular amino acids, which...in turn, are related to circulating levels of amino acids outside of cells. Amino acids are potent inhibitors of autophagy. Autophagy can also be regulated by circulating peptide hormones, which upon receptor binding, presumably trigger signaling cascades involving protein phosphorylation. During starvation, circulating levels of glucagon increase and stimulate autophagy in liver cells. Feeding produces the opposite reaction by increasing the levels of insulin, which in turn, decreases autophagy. Diurnal feeding rhythms cause the numbers of autophagic vacuoles to vary along with the fluctuation of essential amino acids in the blood."

5. Metabolic pathways are required to rebuild the body. Molecules are continuously being built and broken down within cells. In the oxygen-rich environment that we inhabit here on earth, all organic molecules (including proteins, fats, and carbohydrates) may be damaged by nonspecific oxidation mechanisms anywhere in the body. The damage caused by oxidation mechanisms impairs the functions of molecular targets. To overcome the constant damage to molecules caused by oxygen in the body, all molecules in living organisms are re-synthesized on a continual basis, while the damaged molecules are constantly being repaired and recycled.

Because all the enzymes that regulate synthesis and hydrolysis are proteins, it is necessary that the complete set of proteins or "working units" operate at peak performance at all times to maximize repair of the body. The vulnerability in amino acids moving up the food chain therefore has enormous impact on protein health, the balance of positive-charged and negative-charged proteins within the cell. The balance between positive- and negative-charged proteins drives the complete set of metabolic pathways that are required for supercharged health.

6. Medicine has known for more than 30 years that weight loss may be associated with reduced blood pressure, lowered cholesterol and triglycerides, lowered blood sugar, and diminished tendency to develop type II diabetes.

Chapter 12: Strategies for Improving Protein Health

1. A common observation from individuals who take power amino acids is enhanced pep, energy, activity, stamina and endurance. These essential nutrients appear to generate new-found interests in physical activity. They increase both muscle mass and strength. Several subjects showed significant improvements in musculature that led to disappearance of longstanding backaches and even "walking" limps. Each of these benefits were greatly appreciated and led to enthusiastic reviews from study subjects.

Chapter 13: Achieving Successful Weight Control

1. FACTOR4 shakes may be mixed in a shaker cup or bottle with water, soymilk or low-fat milk.
2. FACTOR4 smoothies may be augmented with blackberries, blueberries, strawberries, cranberries, boysenberries, or other berries to vary the taste, color, texture, or nutritional content of Factor4 drinks.
3. Some physicians have questioned the wisdom of replacing two or three meals with dietary supplements on a daily basis. These physicians may be referred to Dr, Nicholas Yphanitides' excellent book, *My Big Fat Greek Diet*. In this book, Dr. Yphanitides explains the personal suffering he endured when he weighed nearly 500 pounds. He explains the nutritional and psychological crusade he conducted during a year's sabbatical

in which he toured America to revel in the national pastime of attending baseball games while dedicating himself to a serious weight loss routine. Shunning all food, even hotdogs and milkshakes in ball stadiums, he existed solely on protein shakes and intense exercise routines for the entire year. His fascinating book details his journey to health while he reduced his body weight from 467 pounds to 195 pounds.

That was 272 pounds of weight lost, or almost three-quarters of a pound a day. And Dr. Yphanitides emerged from his odyssey in good health!

Appendices

"Knowledge and Wisdom, far from being one, have oft-times no connection. Knowledge dwells in heads replete with thoughts of other men, Wisdom in minds attentive to their own. Knowledge is proud that he has learned so much. Wisdom is humble that he knows no more."

– Max Cowper

Appendix I

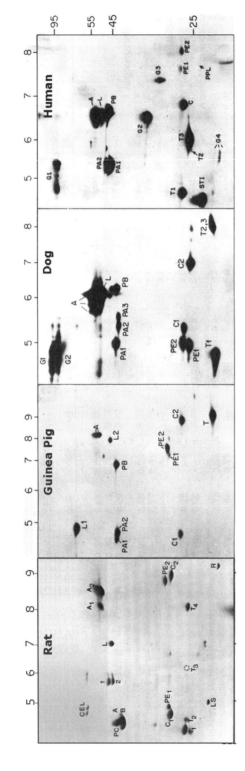

2D Gel Comparison: Pancreatic Digestive Enzymes in 4 Species

218

Comparison of Pancreatic Digestive Enzymes in 5 Species

Protein	Isoelectric points					Apparent molecular weights ($\times 10^{-3}$)				
	Guinea pig	Rat	Rabbit	Dog	Human	Guinea pig	Rat	Rabbit	Dog	Human
Trypsinogen										
1[a]	8.7	4.3	4.6	4.7	4.4	24.4	23.5	25.0	28.0	28.0
2	—	4.4	8.4	8.05	5.5	—	23.5	25.0	26.4	26.0
3	—	8.0	—	8.15	6.4	—	23.5	—	26.4	26.7
Chymotrypsinogen										
1	4.8	4.8	4.8	5.5	7.2	25.8	25.0	26.0	27.5	29.0
2	8.7	9.0	7.1	7.1	—	25.8	25.0	26.5	27.5	—
3	—	—	—	9.5	—	—	—	—	—	—
Proelastase										
1	6.9	4.9	—	5.0	7.6	28.0	26.0	—	29.8	30.5
2	7.5	9.2	—	5.3	7.9	28.0	28.0	—	30.0	30.5
Procarboxypeptidase A										
1	4.6	4.3–4.6	5.0	5.0	4.6	45.0	47–52	47.0	47.3	46.0
2	4.8	—	5.2	5.5	4.7	45.0	—	47.0	45.5	47.0
3	—	—	—	5.7	—	—	—	—	45.5	—
Procarboxypeptidase B										
1	6.6	4.3–4.6	6.2	6.3	6.2	47.7	47–52	47.0	46.7	47.0
2	—	—	—	—	6.7	—	—	—	—	47.0
Prophospholipase A_2										
1	—	—	—	7.3	7.5	—	—	—	—	17.5
α-Amylase										
1	8.4	8.6	6.4	6.0	6.3	52–53	53–55	104.0	53–54	54.8
2	—	8.9	—	—	—	—	—	—	—	—
Lipase										
1	5.0	6.8	6.0	5.9[b]	6.5[b]	66.0	50.0	53.0	55.0[b]	50.5[b]
2	8.1	—	—	—	—	49.7	—	—	—	—
RNase										
1	8.7	9.2	—	—	—	13.0	14.0	—	—	—
2	8.8	—	—	—	—	13.6	—	—	—	—
Glycoprotein										
1	—	—	—	3.9–4.2	3.9	—	—	—	97.0	93.0
2	—	—	—	3.9–4.2	5.2	—	—	—	92.0	36.5
3	—	—	—	—	7.2	—	—	—	—	—
4	—	—	—	—	5.4[c]	—	—	—	—	15.7[c]

[a] Isoenzymic forms are numbered from anode to cathode in accordance with the IUPAC–IUB Commission on biochemical nomenclature of multiple forms of enzymes.
[b] Also demonstrated to be glycoproteins.
[c] Lithostatin.

Appendix II

Publications of George A. Scheele, M.D.

2D Gel Electrophoresis

1. Scheele, G. (1975) Two dimensional gel analysis of soluble proteins—Characterization of guinea pig exocrine pancreatic proteins. *J. Biol. Chem.* 250: 5375–85.
2. Scheele, G, Palade, G, and Tartakoff, A (1978) Cell fractionation studies on the guinea pig pancreas. Redistribution of exocrine proteins during tissue homogenization. *J. Cell Biol.* 78: 110–30.
3. Bieger, W. and Scheele, G. (1980) Two-dimensional isoelectric focusing/sodium dodecyl sulfate gel electrophoresis of protein mixtures containing active or potentially active proteases. Analysis of human exocrine pancreatic proteins, *Anal. Biochem.* 109: 222–230.
4. Scheele, G. (1980) Human pancreatic cancer: Analysis of proteins contained in pancreatic juice by two-dimensional isoelectric focusing/sodium dodecyl sulfate gel electrophoresis. *Cancer,* 47: 1513–15.
5. Scheele, G., Pash, J. and Bieger, W. (1981) Identification of proteins according to biological activity following separation by two-dimensional isoelectric focusing/sodium dodecyl sulfate gel electrophoresis—Analysis of human exocrine pancreatic proteins. *Anal. Biochem.* 112: 304–13.
6. Scheele, G., Bartelt, D. and Bieger, W. (1981) Characterization of human exocrine pancreatic proteins by two-dimensional isoelectric focusing/sodium dodecyl sulfate gel electrophoresis. *Gastroenterology,* 80: 461–73.
7. Rohr, G., Kern, H. and Scheele, G. (1981) Enteropancreatic circulation of digestive enzymes does not exist in the rat. *Nature,* 292: 470–72.
8. Scheele, G. (1981) Analysis of the secretory process in the exocrine pancreas by two-dimensional isoelectric focusing/sodium dodecyl sulfate gel electrophoresis. In *Methods in Cell Biology* (A. Hand and C. Oliver, eds.), 23: 345–58.

9. Scheele, G. and Jacoby, R. (1982) Conformational changes associated with proteolytic processing of presecretory proteins allow glutathione-catalyzed formation of native disulfide bonds. *J. Biol. Chem.* 257, 12277–82.

10. Scheele, G. (1982) Two dimensional electrophoresis in basic and clinical research as exemplified by studies on the exocrine pancreas, *Clin. Chem.*, 28: 1056–61.

11. Rohr, G. and Scheele, G. (1983) Transcellular transport of proteins studied in vivo, In *Methods in Enzymology, Biomembranes* (eds. S. Fleicher and B. Fleicher), 98: 17–27.

12. Rohr, G. and Scheele, G. (1983) Fate of radioactive exocrine pancreatic proteins injected into the blood circulation of the rat. Tissue uptake and transepithelial excretion, *Gastroenterology*, 85: 991–1002.

13. Schick, J., Beil-Moeller, H., Kern, H.F. and Scheele, G.A. (1982) Differential rates of synthesis of individual pancreatic enzymes during prolonged in vivo stimulation, In *Mechanisms of Intestinal Adaptation* (Robinson, JWL, Dowling, RH, Riecken, EO, eds.), MTP Press, pp 511–514.

14. Schick, J., Kern, H. and Scheele, G. (1984) Hormonal stimulation in the exocrine pancreas results in coordinate and anticoordinate regulation of protein synthesis, *J. Cell Biol.* 99: 1559–64.

15. Schick, J., Verspohl, R., Kern, H. and Scheele, G. (1984) Two distinct genetic patterns of response in the exocrine pancreas to inverse changes in protein and carbohydrate in the diet, *Am. J. Physiol.* 248: G611–616.

16. Scheele, G. (1984) Analysis of human exocrine proteins in health and disease by use of two dimensional isoelectric focusing/SDS gel electrophoresis. In *Pancreatitis, Concepts, and Classification* (eds. K. Gyr, M. Singer, and H. Sarles) Elsevier Biomedical Press, pp 89–94

17. Scheele, G. (1986) Two dimensional electrophoresis in the analysis of exocrine pancreatic proteins, *In The Exocrine Pancreas: Biology, Pathobiology and Diseases* (V.L. Go, J.D. Gardner, F.P., Brooks, E. Lebenthal, E.P. DiMagno, G.A. Scheele, eds.) Raven Press. New York, NY, pp 185–192.

18. Scheele, G. (1986) Regulation of gene expression in the exocrine pancreas, In *The Exocrine Pancreas: Biology, Pathobiology and Diseases*

(V.L. Go, J.D. Gardner, F.P., Brooks, E. Lebenthal, E.P. DiMagno, G.A. Scheele, eds.) Raven Press. New York, NY, pp 55–67.

19. Scheele, G. and Tartakoff, A. (1985) Exit of nonglycosylated secretory proteins from the RER is asynchronous in the exocrine pancreas, *J. Biol. Chem.* 260: 926–931.

20. Kern, H., Rausch, U. and Scheele, G. (1986) Pancreatic adaptation to nutritional substrates in the diet is regulated by specific hormones, In *Adaptation in the Small Instestine and Pancreas* (H. Dowling, U. Folsch and E.O. Riecken, eds.) Gut, 28: 89–94.

21. Rausch, U., Vasiloudes, P., Rudiger, K., Kern, H. and Scheele, G. (1986) Lipase synthesis in the rat pancreas is regulated by secretin, *Pancreas*, 1: 522–528.

22. Scheele, G. and Kern H.F. (1989) Selective regulation of gene expression in the exocrine pancreas. *Handbook Physiol., Section 6, The Gastrointestinal System, Vol. III, salivary, gastric, pancreatic and hepatobiliary secretion* (J. Forte, ed.) Oxford University Press, NY, pp 499–513.

23. Lutcke, H., Rausch, U., Vasiloudes, P., Scheele, G.A. and Kern, H.F. (1989) A fourth trypsinogen (P23) in the rat pancreas induced by CCK, *Nuc. Acids Res.*, 17: 6736.

24. Padfield, P.J. and Scheele, G.A. (1993) The use of two-dimensional gel electrophoresis and high performance liquid chromatography for the analysis of pancreatic juice, In *The Pancreas, Biology, Pathobiology and Diseases* (V.L. Go, J.D. Gardiner, H.A. Reber, E. Lebenthal, E.P. DiMagno, G.A. Scheele, eds.) Raven Press, New York, NY pp 265–273.

25. Scheele, G. (1993) Regulation of pancreatic gene expression in response to hormones and nutritional substrates, In *The Pancreas, Biology, Pathobiology and Diseases* (V.L. Go, J.D. Gardiner, H.A. Reber, E. Lebenthal, E.P. DiMagno, G.A. Scheele, eds.) Raven Press, New York, NY pp 103–120.

Pancreatic Function

1. Morris, R.E., Robinson, P.R., and Scheele, G.A. (1964) The relationship of angiotensin to renal hypertension. *Canad. Med. Assn. J.* 90: 272–279.

2. Scheele, G.A. and Kitzes, G. (1969) Analysis of academic training programs in Gastroenterology for the 10 year period 1957–1967, *Gastroenterology,* 57: 203–215.

3. Scheele, G. and Palade, G. (1975) Studies on the pancreas of the guinea pig – parallel discharge of exocrine enzyme activities, *J. Biol. Chem.* 250: 2660–70.

4. Tartakoff, A., Jamieson, J., Scheele, G., and Palade, G. (1975) Studies on the pancreas of the guinea pig—parallel processing and discharge of exocrine protein. *J. Biol. Chem.* 250: 2671–81.

5. Devillers-Thiery, A., Kindt, T., Scheele, G., and Blobel, G. (1975) Homology in the amino-terminal sequence of precursors to pancreatic secretory proteins. *Proc. Nat'l Acad. Sci.,USA,* 72: 5016–20.

6. Haymovits, A. and Scheele, G. (1976) Cellular cyclic nucleotides and enzyme secretion in the pancreatic acinar cell. *Proc. Nat'l Acad. Sci., USA,* 73: 156–60.

7. Scheele, G. (1976) Role of calcium in secretion, In *Proceedings of the Cystic Fibrosis Foundation,* pp 3–4.

8. Scheele, G.A. (1976) Secretory proteins of the exocrine pancreas. In *Cell Biology* (PL Altman and DD Katz, eds., Federation of American Societies for Experimental Biology, Bethesda, MD, pp 334–6.

9. Scheele, G., Dobberstein, B. and Blobel, G. (1978) Transfer of proteins across membranes. Biosynthesis in vitro of pretrypsinogen and trypsinogen by cell fractions of canine pancreas. *Eur. J. Biochem.* 82: 593–9.

10. Scheele, G and Haymovits, A (1978) Calcium dependent discharge of secretory proteins in guinea pig pancreatic lobules. In Calcium Transport and cell Function (eds. A Scarpa and E Carafoli), *Annals of the NY Academy of Sciences,* 307: pp 648–52.

11. Scheele, G and Haymovits, A (1979) Cholinergic and peptide stimulated discharge of secretory proteins in guinea pig pancreatic lobules: Role of intracellular and extracellular calcium, *J. Biol. Chem.* 254: 10346–53.

12. Scheele, G. and Blackburn, P. (1979) Role of the mammalian ribonuclease inhibitor in cell-free protein synthesis. *Proc. Nat'l Acad. Sci.,USA*, 76: 4898–4902.

13. Scheele, G. (1979) The secretory process in the pancreatic exocrine cell, *Mayo Clinic Proceedings*, 54: 420–7.

14. Scheele, G. (1980) Biosynthesis, segregation, and secretion of exportable proteins in the exocrine pancreas. *Am. J. Physiol.* 1: G467–77.

15. Bieger, W and Scheele, G (1980) A sensitive and specific assay for elastase activity using ^{3}H elastin as substrate. *Anal. Biochem.* 104: 239–46.

16. Scheele, G and Haymovits, A (1980) Potassium and ionophore A23187 induced discharge of secretory protein in guinea pig pancreatic lobules: Role of extracellular calcium, *J. Biol. Chem.* 255: 4918–27.

17. Iacino, D., Scheele, G., and Liebow, C. (1980) Secretory response of the rabbit pancreas to cholecystokinin-pancreozymin stimulation, *Am. J. Physiol.* 239: G247–54.

18. Bartelt, D.C. and Scheele, G. (1980) Calmodulin and calmodulin-binding proteins in canine pancreas, *Ann. NY Acad. Sci.*, 356: 356–357

19. Scheele, G., Jacoby, R. and Carne, T. (1980) Mechanism of compartmentation of secretory proteins I. Transport of exocrine pancreatic proteins across the microsomal membrane. *J. Cell Biol.* 87: 611–28.

20. Scheele, G. (1982) Pancreatic zymogen granules, In *The Secretory Granule* (A. Poisner and J. Trifaro, eds.) Elsevier Biomedical Press, pp 213–46.

21. Carne, T. and Scheele, G. (1982) Amino acid sequences of transport peptides associated with canine pancreatic proteins. *J. Biol. Chem.* 257, 4133–40.

22. Scheele, G. and Jacoby, R. (1982) Conformational changes associated with proteolytic processing of presecretory proteins allow glutathione-catalyzed formation of native disulfide bonds. *J. Biol. Chem.* 257, 12277–82.

23. Scheele, G. and Jacoby, R. (1983) Proteolytic processing of presecretory proteins is required for development of biological activities in pancreatic exocrine proteins, *J. Biol. Chem.* 258: 2005–9.

24. Carne, T. and Scheele, G. (1983) The role of presecretory proteins in the secretory process. In *The Secretory Process* (ed. Marc Cantin) Karger Press, Basel, Switzerland, pp 73–101.

25. Scheele, G. (1983) Methods for the study of protein translocation across the RER membrane using the reticulocyte lysate translation system and canine pancreatic microsomal membranes. In *Methods in Enzymology, Biomembranes* (eds. S. Fleicher and B. Fleicher) 96: 94–110.

26. Scheele, G. (1983) pancreatic Lobules in the in vitro study of pancreatic acinar cell function, In *Methods in Enzymology, Biomembranes* (eds. S. Fleicher and B. Fleicher), 98: 17–27.

27. Bartelt, D.C., Carlin, R.C., Scheele, G.A. and Cohen, W.D. (1982) The cytoskeletal system of nucleated erythrocytes, II. Presence of a high molecular weight calmodulin binding protein, *J. Cell Biol.* 95: 278–84.

28. Bartelt, D.D., Carlin, R.K., Scheele, G.A. and Cohen, W.D. (1984) Similarities between the Mr 245,000 calmodulin-binding protein of the dogfish erythrocyte cytoskeleton and alpha-fodrin, *Arch. Biochem. Biophys.* 230: 18–20.

29. Wicker, C., Puigserver, A. and Scheele, G. (1984) Dietary regulation of levels of active mRNA coding for amylase and serine protease zymogens in the rat pancreas, *Eur. J. Biochem.* 139: 381–387.

30. Wicker, C., Scheele, G. and Puigserver, A. (1983) Adaptation au regime alimentaire du niveau des ARNm codant pour l'amylase et les proteases a serine pancreatiques chez le rat, *C. R. Acad. Sc. Paris*, 297: 281–284.

31. Kern, H., Adler, G. and Scheele, G. (1984) Concept of flow and compartmentation in understanding the pathobiology of pancreatitis. In *Pancreatitis, Concepts and Classification* (eds. Gyr, K., Singer, M. and Sarles, H.) Elsevier Biomedical Press, pp 3–9.

32. Scheele, G., Adler, G. and Kern, H. (1984) The role of lysosomes in the development of acute pancreatitis, In *Pancreatitis, Concepts and Classification* (eds. K. Gyr, M. Singer and H. Sarles) Elsevier Biomedical Press, pp 17–23.

33. Kern, H., Warshaw, A. and Scheele, G. (1984) Fine structure of protein precipitations in acinar luminae in the normal human pancreas and in pancreatitis, In *Pancreatitis, Concepts and Classification* (eds. K. Gyr, M. Singer, and H. sarles) Elsevier Biomedical Press, pp 101–105.

34. Scheele, G. (1984) Analysis of human exocrine proteins in health and disease by use of two dimensional isoelectric focusing/SDS gel

electrophoresis. In *Pancreatitis, Concepts, and Classification* (eds. K. Gyr, M. Singer, and H. Sarles) Elsevier Biomedical Press, pp 89–94

35. Scheele, G. (1984) Biochemical concepts and markers in pancreatitis, In *Pancreatitis, Concepts and Classification* (eds. K. Gyr, M. Singer and H. Sarles) Elsevier Biomedical Press, pp 119–125.

36. Kern, H., Adler, G. and Scheele, G. (1985) Structural and biochemical characterization of maximal and supramaximal hormonal stimulation in the rat exocrine pancreas, *Scand. J. Gastroenterology* [Suppl.] 112: 20–29.

37. Scheele, G. (1986) Early biochemical events in the biogenesis and topogenesis of secretory and membrane proteins, In *Molecular and Cellular Biology of Digestion* (P. Desnuelle, H. Sjostrom, and O. Noren, eds.) Elsevier Biomedical Press, pp 43–59.

38. Scheele, G. and Kern, H. (1986) The exocrine pancreas, In *Molecular Cellular Biology of Digestion* (P. Desnuelle, H. Sjostrom, and O. Noren, eds.) Elsevier Biomedical Press, pp 173–194.

39. Adler, G., Kern, H. and Scheele, G. (1986) Experimental models and concepts in acute pancreatitis, In *The Exocrine Pancreas: Biology, Pathobiology and Diseases* (V.L. Go, J.D. Gardner, F.P., Brooks, E. Lebenthal, E.P. DiMagno, G.A. SchBiblioeele, eds.) Raven Press. New York, NY, pp 407–421.

40. Scheele, G. (1986) Cellular processing of proteins in the exocrine pancreas, In *The Exocrine Pancreas: Biology, Pathobiology and Diseases* (V.L. Go, J.D. Gardner, F.P., Brooks, E. Lebenthal, E.P. DiMagno, G.A. Scheele, eds.) Raven Press. New York, NY, pp 69–85.

41. Pitchumoni, C.S., Scheele, G.A., Lee, P.C., Lebenthal, E. (1986) Effects of nutrition on the exocrine pancreas, In *The Exocrine Pancreas: Biology, Pathobiology and Diseases* (V.L. Go, J.D. Gardner, F.P., Brooks, E. Lebenthal, E.P. DiMagno, G.A. Scheele, eds.) Raven Press. New York, NY, pp 387–406.

42. Pinsky, S., LaForge, S., Luc, V. and Scheele, G. (1983) Identification of cDNA clones encoding specific secretory isoenzyme forms; Determination of the primary structure of dog pancreatic prechymotrypsinogen 2 mRNA, *Proc. Nat'l Acad. Sci.,USA*, 80: 7486–7490.

43. Wicker, C., Puigserver, A., Rausch, U., Scheele, G. and Kern, H. (1985) Multiple level caerulein control of the gene expression of secretory proteins in the rat pancreas. *Eur. J. Biochem.* 151: 461–466.

44. Pinsky, S.,LaForge, K. S., and Scheele, G. (1985) Differential regulation of trypsinogen mRNA translation: Full-length mRNA sequences encoding two oppositely charged trypsinogen isoenzymes in the dog pancreas. *Mol. and Cell. Biol.* 5: 2669–2676.

45. Kerfelec, B., LaForge, K.L., Puigserver, A. and Scheele, G. (1986) Primary structures of canine pancreatic lipase and phospholipase A₂ messenger RNAs, *Pancreas*, 1: 430–437.

46. Bartelt, D., Wolff, D. and Scheele, G. (1986) Calmodulin-binding proteins and calmodulin-regulated enzymes in dog pancreas. *Biochem. J.* 240: 753–763.

47. Lutcke, H., Scheele, G. and Kern, H. (1987) Time course and cellular site of mitotic activity in the rat exocrine pancreas during sustained hormone stimulation, *Cell Tiss. Res.*, 247: 364–370.

48. Scheele, G., Adler, G. and Kern, H. (1987) Exocytosis occurs at the lateral plasma membrane of the pancreatic acinar cell during supramaximal secretagogue stimulation, *Gastroenterology*, 92: 345–353.

49. Lutcke, H., Chow, K-C., Mickel, S., Moss, K., Kern, H. and Scheele, G. (1987) Selection of AUG initiation codons differs in plants and animals. *EMBO J.* 6: 43–48.

50. Steinhilber, W., Poensgen, J., Rausch, U., Kern, H. and Scheele, G. (1988) Translational control of anionic trypsinogen and amylase synthesis in rat pancreas in response to caerulein stimulation. *Proc. Nat'l Acad. Sci., USA*, 85: 6597–6601.

51. Wicker, C., Scheele, G.A. and Puigserver, A. (1988) Pancreatic adaptation to dietary lipids is mediated by changes in lipase mRNA. *Biochimie*, 70: 1277–1283.

52. Scheele, G.A. (1988) Molecular sorting of proteins into the cisternal secretory pathway, *Biochimie*, 70: 1269–1276.

53. Swarovsky, B., Steinhilber, W., Scheele, G.A. and Kern, H.F. (1988) Coupled induction of exocrine proteins and intracellular compartments involved in the secretory pathway in AR4–2J cells by glucocorticoids, Eur. *J. Cell Biol.* 47: 101–111.

54. Mickel, F.S., Weidenbach, F., Swarovsky, B., LaForge, K.S., Scheele, G.A. (1989) Structure of the canine pancreatic lipase gene. *J. Biol. Chem.* 264: 12895–12901.

55. Scheele, G. and Kern, H.F. (1989) Cellular compartmentation and protein processing in the exocrine pancreas. *Handbook Physiol., Section*

6, *The Gastrointestinal System, Vol. III, salivary, gastric, pancreatic and hepatobiliary secretion* (J. Forte, ed.) Oxford University Press, NY, pp 477–498.

56. Fukuoka, S.-I. And Scheele, G.A. (1989) Complementary nucleotide sequence for monitor peptide, a novel cholecystokinin-releasing peptide in the rat, *Nuc. Acids Res.* 17: 10111.

57. Fukuoka, S.-I. And Scheele, G.A. (1990) Rapid and selective cloning of monitor peptide, a novel CCK-releasing peptide, using minimal amino acid sequence and the polymerase chain reaction. *Pancreas*, 5: 1–7.

58. Kerfelec, B., LaForge, K.S., Vasiloudes, P., Puigserver, A. and Scheele, G. (1990) Isolation and sequence of the canine pancreatic phospholipase A_2 gene, *Eur. J. Biochem.*, 190: 299–304.

59. Fukuoka, S.-I., Taniguchi, Y., Kitigawa, Y. and Scheele, G.A. (1990) Full-length cDNA sequence encoding canine pancreatic colipase, *Nuc. Acids Res.*, 18: 5549.

60. Fukuoka, S.-I. And Scheele, G.S. (1990) Nucleotide sequence encoding the major glycoprotein (GP2) of rat pancreatic secretory (zymogen) granule membranes. *Nuc. Acids Res.* 18: 5900.

61. Fukuoka, S.-I., Freedman, S.D. and Scheele, G.A. (1991) A single gene encodes membrane bound and free forms of GP-2, the major glycoprotein in pancreatic secretory (zymogen) granule membranes. *Proc. Nat'l Acad. Sci., USA*, 88: 2898–2902.

62. Leach, S.D., Modlin, I.M., Scheele, G.A. and Gorelick, F.S. (1991) Intracellular activation of digestive zymogens in rat pancreatic acini, Stimulation by high doses of cholecystokinin, *J. Clin. Invest.* 87: 362–366.

63. Fukuoka, S.-I. And Scheele, G.A. (1991) Novel strategy for synthesis of full-length double-stranded cDNA transcripts without dC-dG tails. *Nuc. Acids Res.* 19: 6961–6962.

64. Fukuoka, S.-I., Freedman, S.D., Yu, H., Sukhatme, V. and Scheele, G.A. (1992) GP2/THP gene family encodes self-binding GPI-linked proteins in apical vesicular membranes of pancreas and kidney, *Proc. Nat'l Acad. Sci.,USA*, 89: 1189–1193.

65. Freedman, S.D., and Scheele, G.A. (1993) Regulated secretory proteins in the exocrine pancreas aggregate under conditions that mimic the trans-Golgi network, *Biochem. Biophys. Res. Comm.* 2: 992–999.

66. Pitchumoni, C.S. and Scheele, G.A. (1993) Interdependence of nutrition and exocrine pancreatic function, In *The Pancreas, Biology, Pathobiology and Diseases* (V.L. Go, J.D. Gardiner, H.A. Reber, E. Lebenthal, E.P. DiMagno, G.A. Scheele, eds.) Raven Press, New York, NY pp 449–473.

67. Scheele, G.A. and Kern, H.F. (1993) Cellular compartmentation, protein processing and secretion in the exocrine pancreas, In *The Pancreas, Biology, Pathobiology and Diseases* (V.L. Go, J.D. Gardiner, H.A. Reber, E. Lebenthal, E.P. DiMagno, G.A. Scheele, eds.) Raven Press, New York, NY pp 121–150.

68. Fukuoka, S.I., Zhang, D.-E., Taniguchi, Y. and Scheele, G.A. (1993) Structure of the pancreatic colipase gene includes two protein binding sites in the promoter region, *J. Biol. Chem.* 11312–11320.

69. Freedman, S.D. and Scheele, G.A. (1993) Reversible pH-induced homophilic binding of GP2, a glycosyl-phosphatidylinositol-anchored protein in pancreatic zymogen granule membranes. Eur. *J. Cell Biol.* 61: 229–238.

70. Scheele, G.A. (1993) Extracellular and intracellular messengers in diet-induced regulation of pancreatic gene expression, In *Physiology of the Gastrointestinal Tract* (L.R. Johnson, ed.) Raven Press, New York, NY,

71. Freedman, S.D. Sakamoto, K. and Scheele, G.A. (1993) Nonparallel secretion of GP2, a GPI-linked protein in exocrine pancreas, implies luminal coupling reactions between acinar and duct cells, *Am. J. Physiol.*, 267: G40–G51.

72. Wada, I., Ou, W. J. Lew, M.C., Scheele, G.A. (1994) Chaperone function of calnexin for the folding intermediate of gp80, the major secretory protein in MDCK cells, *J. Biol. Chem.* 269: 7464–7472.

73. Freedman, S.D. and Scheele, G.A. (1994) Acid-Base interactions during exocrine pancreatic secretion. Primary role for ductal bicarbonate in acinar lumen function. *Annals NY Acad. Sci.* 713: 199–206.

74. Scheele, G.A., Fukuoka, S.-I., Freedman, S.D. (1994) Role of the GP2/THP family of GPI-anchored proteins in membrane trafficking during regulated exocrine secretion. *Pancreas*, 9: 139–149.

75. Freedman, S.D., Kern, H.F. and Scheele, G.A. (1994) Apical membrane trafficking during regulated pancreatic exocrine secretion—Role of alkaline pH in the acinar lumen and enzymatic cleavage of GP2, a GPI-linked protein, Eur. *J. Cell Biol.* 65: 354–365.

76. Bimmler, D., Frick, T.W. and Scheele, G.A. (1995) High level secretion of native rat pancreatic lithostatine in a baculovirus expression system, *Pancreas*, 11: 63–76.

77. Scheele, G.A., Fukuoka, S.-I., Kern, H.F. and Freedman, S.D. (1996) Pancreatic dysfunction in cystic fibrosis occurs as a result of impairment in luminal pH, apical trafficking of zymogen granule membranes, and solubilization of secretory enzymes. *Pancreas*, 1: 1–9.

78. Bimmler, D., Graf, R., Scheele, G.A. and Frick, T.W. (1997) Pancreatic stone protein (lithostathine), a physiologically relevant pancreatic calcium crystal inhibitor? *J. Biol. Chem.* 272: 3073–82.

79. Freedman, S.D., Scheele, G.A. and Kern, H.F. (1997) Coupling of ductal and acinar cell function in the exocrine pancreas: novel insights into CF. *Pediatric Pulmonology*, [Suppl. 14] 24: 114–115.

80. Gorelick, F.S., Schmid, S.W., Tang, L.H., Rhee, S., Nathanson, M., Scheele, G.A., Modlin, I.M. (1998) Telenzepine-sensitive muscarinic receptors on the pancreatic acinar cell, *Am. J. Physiol.* 274: G734–41.

81. Freedman, S.D., Kern, H.F. and Scheele, G.A. (1998) Acinar lumen pH regulates endocytosis, but not exocytosis, at the apical plasma membrane of pancreatic acinar cells, Eur. *J. Cell Biol.*, 75: 153–162.

82. Freedman, S.D., Kern, H.F. and Scheele, G.A. (1998) Cleavage of GPI-anchored proteins from the plasma membrane activates apical endocytosis in pancreatic acinar cells, Eur. *J. Cell Biol.*, 75: 163–173.

83. Bimmler, D., Angst, E., Valeri, F., Bain, M., Scheele, G.A., Frick, T.W. and Graf, R. (1999) Regulation of PSP/*reg* in Rat Pancreas: Immediate and Steady State Adaptation to Different Diets, *Pancreas*, 19: 255–267.

84. Graf, R., Schiesser, M., Scheele, G.A., Marquardt, K., Frick, T.W., Ammann, R. and Bimmler, D. (2001) A Family of 16-kDa Pancreatic Secretory Stress Proteins Form Highly Organized Fibrillar Structures upon Tryptic Activation. *J. Biol. Chem.*, 276: 21028–21038.

85. Freedman, S.D., Kern, H.F. and Scheele, G.A. (2001) Pancreatic Acinar Cell Dysfunction in CFTR-/- Mice is Associated with Impairments in Luminal pH and Endocytosis at the Apical Plasma Membrane. *Gastroenterology*, 121: 950–957.

86. Graf, R., Schiesser, M., Lussi, A., Went, P., Scheele, G.A. Bimmler, D. (2002) Coordinate Regulation of Secretory Stress Proteins (PSP/

reg and PAPI, PAPII & PAPIII in the Rat Exocrine Pancreas During Experimental Acute Pancreatitis. *J Surg Res.*: 105(2):136–44.

87. Bimmler, D., Schiesser, M., Perren, A., Scheele, G., Angst, E., Meili, S., Ammann R. and Graf R. (2004) Coordinate Regulation of PSP/reg and PAP Isoforms as a Family of Secretory Stress Proteins in an Animal Model of Chronic Pancreatitis. *J Surg Res*: 118(2), 122–35.

Bibliography

1. Agatston, A. 2003. The *South Beach Diet*. Emmaus, Pa.: Rodale Press.
2. Ahrens, E. H., Jr. 1985. "The Diet-Heart Question in 1985: Has It Really Been Settled?" *Lancet*. May II; 325 (8437):1085–87.
3. —. 1979a. "Dietary Fats and Coronary Heart Disease: Unfinished Business." *Lancet*.
4. Dec. 22/29; 314(8156–57):1345–48.
5. —. 1979b. "Introduction." *American Journal of Clinical Nutrition* 32 (suppl.):2627–31.
6. —. 1957. "Nutritional Factors and Serum Lipid Levels." *American Journal of Medicine*. Dec.; 23(6):928–52.
7. Ahrens, E. H., Jr., J.Hirsch, W. Insult Jr., T. T. Tsaltas, R. Blomstrand, and M. L. Peterson. 1957. "Dietary Control of Serum Lipids in Relation to Atherosclerosis." *JAMA*. Aug. 24; 164 (17):1905–11.
8. Ahrens, E. H., Jr., J. Hirsch, K. Oette, J. W. Farquhar, and Y. Stein. 1961. "Carbohydrate Induced and Fat-Induced Lipemia." *Transactions of the Medical Society of London*. 74:134–46.
9. Ahrens, E. H., Jr., W. Insull. Jr., R. Blomstrand, J. Hirsch, T. T. Tsaltas, and M. L. Peterson. 1957. "The Influence of Dietary Fats on Serum-Lipid Levels in Man." *Lancet*. May II; 272 (6976):943–53.
10. Akinyanju, P. A., R. U. Qureshi, A. J. Salter, and J. Yudkin. 1968. "Effect of an 'Atherogenic' Diet Containing Starch or Sucrose on the Blood Lipids of Young Men." *Nature*. June 8; 218 (5145):975–77.
11. Albrink, M. J. 1965. "Diet and Cardiovascular Disease." *Journal of the American Dietetic Association*. Jan.; 46: 26–29.
12. —. 1963. "The Significance of Serum Triglycerides." *Journal of the American Dietetic Association*. Jan.; 42:29–31.
13. —. 1962. "Triglycerides, Lipoproteins, and Coronary Artery Disease." *Archives of Internal Medicine*. 109(3):345–59.
14. Albrink, M. J., P. H. Lavietes, E. B. Man, and J. R. Paul. 1962. "Relationship Between Serum Lipids and the Vascular Complications

of Diabetes from 1931 to 1961." *Transactions of the Association of American Physicians. 75:235–41.*

15. Albrink, M. J., and J. W. Meigs. 1965. "The Relationship Between Serum Triglycerides and Skinfold Thickness in Obese Subjects." *Annals of the New York Academy of Sciences.* Oct. 8; 131 (1):673–83.

16. American Diabetes Association (ADA). 2006. "Nutrition Recommendations and Interventions for Diabetes—2006: A Position Statement of the American Diabetes Association." *Diabetes Care.* Sept.; 29(9):214–57.

17. —. 1971. "Principles of Nutrition and Dietary Recommendations for Patients with Diabetes Mellitus: 1971." *Diabetes.* Sept.; 20(9):633–34.

18. American Heart Association [AHA]. 2005. *The No-Fad Diet: A Personal Plan for Healthy Weight Loss.* New York: Clarkson Potter.

19. Anderson, J. H. 1935. "The Treatment of Obesity." *Lancet.* Sept. 14; 226(5846):604–8.

20. Anderson, J. H:, A. Keys, and F. Grande. 1957. "'The Effects of Different Food Fats on Serum Cholesterol Concentration in Man." *Journal of Nutrition.* July 10; 62(3):421–24.

21. Anderson, J. T., A. Lawler, and A. Keys. 1957. "Weight Gain from Simple Overeating. 2. Serum Lipids and Blood Volume." *Journal of Clinical Investigation. 36(1):81–88.*

22. Anderson, K. M., W. P. Castelli, and D. Levy. 1987. "Cholesterol and Mortality: 30 Years of Follow-Up from the Framingham Study." *JAMA.* April 24; 257(16):2176–80.

23. Anon. 1988. "Report of the National Cholesterol Education Program Expert Panel on Detection, Evaluation, and Treatment of High Blood Cholesterol in Adults: The Expert Panel." *Archives of Internal Medicine.* Jan.; 148(1):36–69.

24. —. 1984b. "Lowering Blood Cholesterol to Prevent Heart Disease." NIH Consensus Development Conference December 10–12, 1984. Program and Abstracts. National Heart, Lung, and Blood Institute and the NIH Office of Medical Applications of Research.

25. —. 1983. "This Week's Citation Classic—Stunkard A. & McLaren-Hume M. 'The Results of Treatment for Obesity: A Review of the Literature and Report of a Series.' " *Current Content.* Nov. 23; 67(21):24.

26. —. 1973. "A Critique of Low-Carbohydrate Ketogenic Weight Reduction Regimens: A Review of 'Dr. Atkins' Diet Revolution.'" *JAMA*. June 4; 224(10):1415–19.

27. —. 1969. *White House Conference on Food, Nutrition, and Health: Final Report*. Washington, D.C.: U.S. Government Printing Office.

28. —. 1967. "Coronary Heart Disease and Carbohydrate Metabolism." *JAMA*. Sept. 25; 201(13):164–65.

29. —. 1966. "Blake Donaldson, Internist, Author." *New York Times*. Feb. 21; 39.

30. —. 1950. "Why Executives Drop Dead." *Fortune*. June; 41:88–91,149–56.

31. —. 1930a. "All-Meat Eskimo Diet Is Declared Harmful by University of Michigan Doctors After Test." *New York Times*. March 17; 15.

32. Armstrong, B. K. 1977. "The Role of Diet in Human Carcinogenesis with Special Reference to Endometrial Cancer." In Hiatt, Watson, and Winsten, eds., 1977, 557–65.

33. Armstrong, B. K., and R. Doll. 1975. "Environmental Factors and Cancer Incidence and Mortality in Different Countries with Special Reference to Dietary Practices." *International Journal of Cancer*. *15:617–31.*

34. Amer, P., and R. H. Eckel. 1998. "Adipose Tissue as a Storage Organ." In Bray, Bouchard, and James, eds., 1998, 379–96.

35. Arner, P., P. Engfeldt, and H. Lithell. 1981. "Site Differences in the Basal Metabolism of Subcutaneous Fat in Obese Women." *Journal of Clinical Endocrinology & Metabolism*. Nov.; 53(5):948–52.

36. Ashworth, A, R. Bell, W. P. James, and J. C. Waterlow. 1968. "Calorie Requirements of Children Recovering from Protein-Calorie Malnutrition." *Lancet*. Sept. 14; 2.92.(7568):600–603.

37. Astwood, E. B. 1962. "The Heritage of Corpulence." *Endocrinology*. Aug.; 71:337–41. Atkins, R. C. 1973- Prepared Statement of Dr. Robert C. Atkins. In Select Committee on Nutrition and Human Needs of the United States Senate 1973b, 4–8.

38. —. 1972. *Dr. Atkins' Diet Revolution: The High Calorie Way to Stay Thin Forever*. New York: David McKay.

39. Aykroyd, W. R. 1967. *The Story of Sugar*. Chicago: Quadrangle Books.

40. Azar, G. J., and W. L. Bloom. 1963. "Similarities of Carbohydrate Deficiency and Fasting. II. Ketones, Nonesterified Fatty Acids and Nitrogen Excretion." *Archives of Internal Medicine*. Sept.; 112:338–4.

41. Babkin, B.P. 1949. *Pavlov, A Biography*. The University of Chicago Press.

42. Bailar, J. C., 3rd. 1980. "Cause and Effect in Epidemiology: What Do We Know About Hypertriglyceridemia?" *New England Journal of Medicine*. June 19; 302(25):1417–18. Baker, B. M., I. D. Frantz, Jr., A. Keys, et al. 1963. "The National Diet-Heart Study: An Initial Report." *JAMA*. July 13; 185:105–6.

43. Ballard-Barbash, R. 1999. "Energy Balance, Anthropometry, and Cancer." In *Nutritional Oncology*, ed. D. Heber, G. L. Blackburn, and V. L. Go (San Diego: Academic Press), 137–52.

44. Bantle, J. P., D. C. Laine, G. W. Castle, J. W. Thomas, B. J. Hoogwerf, and F. C. Goetz. 1983. "Postprandial Glucose and Insulin Responses to Meals Containing Different Carbohydrates in Normal and Diabetic Subjects." *New England Journal of Medicine*. July 7; 309(1):7–12.

45. Bantle, J. P., J. Wylie-Rosett, A. L. Albright, et al. 2006. "Nutrition Recommendations and Interventions for Diabetes—2006: A Position Statement of the American Diabetes Association." *Diabetes Care*. Sept.; 29(9):2140–45.

46. Bartke, A. 2002. "Insulin-Like Growth Factor I and Mammalian Aging." *Science of Aging Knowledge Environment*. April 24; 2002(16):VP4. Online at httoP//sageke.sciencemag.org/cgi/content/full/sageke;2002/16/VP4.

47. Baserga, R. 2004. "Targeting the IGF-I Receptor: From Rags to Riches." *European Journal of Cancer*. Sept.; 40(14):2013–15.

48. Baserga, R., F. Peruzzi, and K. Reiss. 2003. "The IGF-I Receptor in Cancer Biology." *International Journal of Cancer*. Dec. 20; 107(6):873–77.

49. Bauer, J. 1945. *Constitution and Disease: Applied Constitutional Pathology*. New York: Grone & Stratton.

50. —. 1941. "Obesity: Its Pathogenesis, Etiology, and Treatment: *Archives of Internal Medicine*. May; 67(5):968–94.

51. —. 1940. "Observations on Obese Children." *Archives of Pediatrics*. 57:631–40

52. Beaglehole, R., M. A. Foulkes, I. A. Prior, and E. F. Eyles. 1980. "Cholesterol and Mortality in New Zealand Maoris: *British Medical Journal*. Feb. 2; 280(6210):285–87.

53. Beaumont, W. 1980. *Experiments and Observations on the Gastric Juice and the Physiology of Digestion*. Birmingham: The Classics of Medicine Library, a Division of Gryphon Editions, Ltd. [First edition published in Plattsburgh, by F.P. Allen in 1833.]

54. Beck, M. 1990. "The Losing Formula." *Newsweek*. April 30; 52. Becker, M. H. 1987. "The Cholesterol Saga: Whither Health Promotion?" *Annals of Internal Medicine*. April; 106(4):623–26.

55. Benedict, F. G. 1925. "The Measurement and Significance of Metabolism," In *Lectures on Nutrition* (Philadelphia: W. B. Saunders), 17–58.

56. Benedict, F. G., and T. M. Carpenter. 1910. *The Metabolism and Energy Transformations of Healthy Man During Rest*. Washington, D.C.: Carnegie Institution of Washington.

57. Benedict, F. G., and L. E. Emmes. 1915. "A Comparison of the Basal Metabolism of Normal Men and Women." *Journal of Biology and Chemistry. 20(3):253–62.*

58. Benedict, F. G., W. R. Miles, P. Roth, and H. M. Smith. 1919. *Human Vitality and Efficiency Under Prolonged Restricted Diet*. Washington, D.C.: Carnegie Institution of Washington.

59. Bennett, W., and J. Gurin. 1982. *The Dieter's Dilemma: Eating Less and Weighing More*. New York: Basic Books.

60. Bernard, C. 1980. *An Introduction to the Study of Experimental Medicine*. Birmingham: The Classics of Medicine Library, a Division of Gryphon Editions, Ltd. [English translation originally published by the MacMillan Company in 1927.]

61. Berneis, K. K., and R. M. Krauss. 2002. "Metabolic Origins and Clinical Significance of LDL Heterogeneity: *journal of Lipid Research*. Sept.; 43(9):1363–79.

62. Berson, S. A., and R. S. Yalow. 1970. "Insulin 'Antagonists' and Insulin Resistance: In *Diabetes Mellitus: Theory and Practice,* ed. M. Ellenberg and H. Rifkin (New York: McGraw.Hill),388–423.

63. —. 1965. "Some Current Controversies in Diabetes Research." *Diabetes*. Sept.; 14(9):549–72.

64. Bertrand, H. A., F. T. Lynd, E. J. Masoro, and B. P. Yu. 1980. "Changes in Adipose Tissue Mass and Cellularity Through Adult Life of Rats Fed ad Libitum or a Life.Prolonging Restricted Diet." *Journal of Gerontology.* Nov.; 35(6):827–35.

65. Bishop, J. E. 1982. "Heart Attacks: A Test Collapses." Wall *Street Journal.* Oct. 6; 32.

66. —. 1961. "Helping the Heart: Major Research Effort Started to See If Diet Can Prevent Attacks." Wall *Street Journal.* Oct. 27; I.

67. Bjorntorp, P. 1985. "Adipose Tissue in Obesity: In Hirsch and Van ltallie, eds., 1985, 163–70.

68. —. 1976. "Effects of Physical Conditioning in Obesity." In Bray, ed., 1976b, 397–406.

69. Bjorntorp, P., M. Cairella, and A. N. Howard, eds. 1981. *Recent Advances in Obesity Research: III.* London: John Libbey.

70. Blackburn, H. n.d. "Ancel Keys: An Appreciation." Online at http:// mbbnet.umn.edu/firsts/blackburn_h.html.

71. —. 1975. "Contrasting Professional Views on Atherosclerosis and Coronary Disease." *New England Journal of Medicine.* Jan. 9; 292(2):105–7.

72. Blackburn, H., and D. R. Jacobs, Jr. 1989. "The Ongoing Natural Experiment of Cardiovascular Diseases in Japan." *Circulation.* March; 79(3):718–20.

73. Blakeslee, A., and J. Stamler. 1966. *Your Heart Has Nine Lives: Nine Steps to Heart Health.* New York: Pocket Books.

74. Bleiler, R. E., E. S. Yearick, S. S. Schnur, I. L. Singson, and M. A. Ohlson. 1963. "Seasonal Variation of Cholesterol in Serum of Men and Women." *American Journal of Clinical Nutrition.* Jan.; 12:12–16.

75. Bliss, M. 1982. *The Discovery of Insulin.* Toronto: McClelland & Stewart.

76. Bloom, W. L., and G. J. Azar. 1963. "Similarities of Carbohydrate Deficiency and Fasting. I. Weight Loss, Electrolyte Excretion, and Fatigue." *Archives of Internal Medicine.* Sept.; 112:333–37.

77. Bluher, M., B. B. Kahn, and C. R. Kahn. 2003. "Extended Longevity in Mice Lacking the Insulin Receptor in Adipose Tissue." *Science.* Jan. 24; 299(5606):572–74.

78. Blundell, J. E., and R. J. Stubbs. 1998. "Diet Composition and the Control of Food Intake." In Bray, Bouchard, and James, eds., 1998, 243–72.

79. Bodkin, N. L., J. S. Hannah, H. K. Ortrneyer, and B. C. Hansen. 1993. "Central Obesity in Rhesus Monkeys: Association with Hyperinsulinemia, Insulin Resistance and Hypertriglyceridemia?" *International Journal of Obesity and Related Metabolic Disorders.* Jan.; 17(1):53–61.

80. Boodman, S. G. 1998. "The First Line of Defense: Those Old Standbys, Diet and Exercise, Are Key Weapons in the Fight Against Cancer." *Washington Post.* Feb. 10; Z25.

81. Bouchard, C., A. Tremblay, J. P. Despres, et al. 1990. "The Response to Long-Term Over-feeding in Identical Twins." *New England Journal of Medicine.* May 24; 322(21):1477–82.

82. Bravata, D. M., L. Sanders, J. Huang, et al. 2003. "Efficacy and Safety of Low Carbohydrate Diets: A Systematic Review." *JAMA.* April 9; 289(14):1837–50.

83. Bray, G. A. 1998. "Classification and Evaluation of the Overweight Patient." In Bray, Bouchard, and James, eds., 1998, 831–54.

84. —. ed. 1980. *Obesity: Comparative Methods of Weight Control.* Westport, Conn.: Tech-nomic Publishing.

85. Bray. G. A.. and J. E. Bethune. eds. 1974. *Treatment and Management of Obesity.* New York: Harper & Row.

86. Bray. G. A.. C. Bouchard. and W. P. James. eds. 1998. *Handbook of Obesity.* New York: Marcel Dekker.

87. Bray. G. A.. S. J. Nielsen. and B. M. Popkin. 2004. "Consumption of High-Fructose Com Syrup in Beverages May Play a Role in the Epidemic of Obesity." *American Journal of Clinical Nutrition.* April; 79(4):537–43.

88. Bray. G. A.. and B. M. Popkin. 1999. "Dietary Fat Affects Obesity Rate." *American Journal of Clinical Nutrition.* Oct.; 70(4):572–73.

89. Brehm. B. J.. R. J. Seeley. S. R. Daniels. and D. A. D'Alessio. 2003. "A Randomized Trial Comparing a Very Low Carbohydrate Diet and a Calorie-Restricted Low Fat Diet on Body Weight and Cardiovascular Risk Factors in Healthy Women." *Journal of Clinical Endocrinology and Metabolism.* April; 88(4):1617–23.

90. Broad. W. J. 1980 Academy Says Curb on Cholesterol Not Needed." *Science.* June 20; 208 (445°):1354–5.

91. Brobeck. J. R. 1993. "Remembrance of Experiments Almost Forgotten." *Appetite.* Dec.; 21(3):225–31.

92. Brody, J. E. 2004a. "Sane Weight Loss in a Carb-Obsessed World: High Fiber and Low Fat." *New York Times.* May 23; F7.

93. —. 2004b. "For Unrefined Healthfulness: Whole Grains." *New York Times.* March 4; F5.

94. —. 1999b. "Doubts Fail to Deter 'The Diet Revolution.' " *New York Times.* May 25; F7.

95. —. 1985. *Jane Brody's Good Food Book: Living the High-Carbohydrate Way.* New York: W. W. Norton.

96. —. 1981a. *Jane Brody's Nutrition Book.* New York: W. W. Norton.

97. Brooks, P. C., R. L. Klemke, S. Schon, J. M. Lewis, M. A. Schwartz, and D. A. Cheresh. 1997. "Insulin-Like Growth Factor Receptor Cooperates with Integrin aVb5 to Promote Tumor Cell Dissemination in Vivo." *Journal of Clinical Investigation.* March; 99(6):1390–98.

98. Brown, E. G., and M. A. Ohlson. 1946. "Weight Reduction of Obese Women of College Age. I. Clinical Results and Basal Metabolism." *Journal of the American Dietetic Association.22:849–57.*

99. Brown, M. S., and J. L. Goldstein. 1985. "A Receptor-Mediated Pathway for Cholesterol Homeostasis." Online at http://nobelprize. org/nobel_prizes/medicine/laureates/1985/brown-lecture.html.

100. Brownell, K. D., and K. B. Horgen. 2004. *Food Fight: The Inside Story of the Food Industry, America's Obesity Crisis, and What We Can Do About It.* New York: McGraw-Hill.

101. Browner, W. S., J. Westenhouse, and J. A. Tice. 1991. "What If Americans Ate Less Fat? A Quantitative Estimate of the Effect on Mortality." *JAMA.* June 26; 265(24):3285–91.

102. Bruch, H. 1973. *Eating Disorders: Obesity, Anorexia Nervosa, and the Person Within.* New York: Basic Books.

103. Bucala, R., Z. Makita, T. Koschinsky, A. Cerami, and H. Vlassara. 1993. "Lipid Advanced Glycosylation: Pathway for Lipid Oxidation in Vivo." *Proceedings of the National Academy of Sciences.* July 15; 90(14): 6434–38.

104. Bunn, H. F., K. H. Gabbay, and P. M. Gallop. 1978. "The Glycosylation of Hemoglobin: Relevance to Diabetes Mellitus." *Science.* April 7; 200(4337):21–27.

105. Bunn, H. F., and P. J. Higgins. 1981. "Reaction of Monosaccharides with Proteins: Possible Evolutionary Significance." *Science.* July 10; 213(4504):222–24.

106. Burkitt, D. P. I99Ia. In interview with Max Blythe, Gloucestershire, 29 October 1991, Interview IV. Royal College of Physicians and Oxford Brookes Medical Sciences Video Archive (MSVA 64).

107. —. I99Ib. In interview with Max Blythe, Gloucestershire, 26 February 1991, Interview III. The Royal College of Physicians and Oxford Brookes Medical Sciences Video Archive (MSVA 64).

108. —. I979a. *Don't Forget Fibre in Your Diet.* London: Martin Dunitz Ltd.

109. Burkitt, D. P., and H. C. Trowell, eds. 1975. *Refined Carbohydrate Foods and Disease: Some Implications of Dietary Fibre.* New York: Academic Press.

110. Burland, W. L., P. D. Samuel, and J. Yudkin, eds. 1974. *Obesity.* New York: Churchill Livingstone.

111. Burroughs. K. D.. S. E. Dunn. J. C. Barrett. and J. A. Taylor. 1999. "Insulin-Like Growth

112. Factor-I: A Key Regulator of Human Cancer Risk?" *Journal of the National Cancer*

113. *Institute.* April 7; 91(7):579–81.

114. Byers. T.. M. Nestle. A. McTiernan. et al. (American Cancer Society 2002 Nutrition and Physical Activity Guidelines Advisory Committee). 2002. "American Cancer Society Guidelines on Nutrition and Physical Activity for Cancer Prevention: Reducing the Risk of Cancer with Healthy Food Choices and Physical Activity." CA: A *Cancer journal for Clinicians.* March–April; 52(2):92–II9.

115. Cahill. G. F.. Jr. 1978. "Obesity and Diabetes." In Bray. ed. 1978. 101–10.

116. —. 1975. "Weight Reduction Diets." In Bray. ed.. 1975. 58–59.

117. —. 1971. "The Banting Memorial Lecture: Physiology of Insulin in Man." *Diabetes.* Dec.; 20(12):785–99.

118. Cahill. G. F.. Jr.. B. Jeanrenaud. B. Leboeuf. and A. E. Renold. 1959. "Effects of Insulin on Adipose Tissue." *Annals of the New York Academy of Sciences.* Sept. 25; 82: 4303-II.

119. Cahill. G. F.. Jr.. and A. E. Renold. 1965. "Regulation of Adipose Tissue Metabolism Within the Intact Organism." In Renold and Cahill. eds.. 1965. 681–84.

120. Cahill. G. F.. Jr.. and R. L. Veech. 2003. "Ketoacids? Good Medicine?" *Transactions of the American Clinical Climatological Association.* II4: 149–61.

121. Campbell. G. D. 1963. "Diabetes in Asians and Africans in and Around Durban." *South African Medical journal.* Nov. 30; 37:1995–208.

122. Carney. R. N.. and A. P. Goldberg. 1984. "Weight Gain After Cessation of Cigarette Smoking: A Possible Role for Adipose-Tissue Lipoprotein Lipase." *New England Journal of Medicine.* March 8; 310(10):614–16.

123. Castelli, W. P., J. T. Doyle, T. Gordon, et al. 1977. "HDL Cholesterol and Other Lipids in Coronary Heart Disease: The Cooperative Lipoprotein Phenotyping Study." *Circulation.* May; 55(5):767–72.

124. Castetter, E. F., and W. H. Bell. 1942. *Pima and Papago Indian Agriculture.* Albuquerque: University of New Mexico Press.

125. Centers for Disease Control and Prevention. 2005. *National Diabetes Fact Sheet: General Information and National Estimates on Diabetes in the United States,* 2005. Atlanta, Ga.: U.S. Department of Health and Human Services, Centers for Disease Control and Prevention.

126. —. 2001. "Physical Activity Trends-United States, 1990–1998." *Morbidity and Mortality Weekly Reports.* March 9; 50(9):166–69. Online at http://www.cdc.gov/mmwr/preview/mmwrhtml/mm5009a3.htrn.

127. Cerami, A., H. Vlassara, and M. Brownlee. 1987. "Glucose and Aging." *Scientific American.* May; 256(5):90–96.

128. Chait, A., J. D. Brunzell, M. A. Denke, et al. 1993. "Rationale of the Diet-Heart Statement of the American Heart Association: Report of the Nutrition Committee," *Circulation.* Dec.; 88(6):3008–29.

129. Chajek-Shaul, T., E. M. Berry, E. Ziv, et al. 1990. "Smoking Depresses Adipose Lipoprotein Lipase Response to Oral Glucose." *European Journal of Clinical Investigation.* June; 20(3):299–304.

130. Chan, J. M., M. J. Stampfer, E. Giovannucci, et al. 1998. "Plasma Insulin-Like Growth Factor-I and Prostate Cancer Risk: A Prospective Study." *Science.* Jan. 23; 279(5350): 563–66.

131. Chen, J., T. C. Campbell, J. Li, and R. Peto. 1990. *Diet, Lifestyle, and Mortality in China: A Study of Characteristics of 65 Chinese Counties.* Joint publication: Oxford University Press; Ithaca, N.Y.: Cornell University Press; and Beijing: People's Medical Publishing House.

132. Cioffi, L. A., W. P. James, and T. B. Van ltallie, eds. 1981. The *Body Weight Regulatory System: Normal and Disturbed Mechanisms.* New York: Raven Press.

133. Clancy, D. J., D. Gems, L. G. Harshman, et al. 2001. "Extension of Life-Span by Loss of CHICO, a Drosophila Insulin Receptor Substrate Protein." *Science.* April 6; 292(5514):104–6.

134. Clarke. H. T. 1941. "Rudolf Schoenheimer." *Science.* Dec. 12; 94(2450):553–54.

135. Cleave, T. L. 1975. The *Saccharine Disease:* The *Master Disease of Our Time.* New Canaan, Conn.: Keats Publishing.

136. Cleave, T. L., and G. D. Campbell. 1966. *Diabetes, Coronary* Thrombosis, *and the Saccharine Disease.* Bristol: John Wright & Sons.

137. Cohen, A. M. 1963. "Effect of Environmental Changes on Prevalence of Diabetes and of Atherosclerosis in Various Ethnic Groups in Israel." In The *Genetics of* Migrant *and Isolate Populations,* ed. E. Goldschmidt. New York: Williams & Wilkins, 127-30.

138. Cohen, A. M., S. Bavly, and R. Poznanski. 1961. "Change of Diet of Yemenite Jews in Relation to Diabetes and Ischaemic Heart-Disease." *Lancet.* Dee. 23; 278(7217):1399–1401.

139. Cohen, B. M. 1954. "Diabetes Mellitus Among Indians of the American Southwest: Its Prevalence and Clinical Characteristics in a Hospitalized Population." *Annals of Internal Medicine.* March; 40(3):588–99.

140. Cohen, M. N. 1989. *Health and the Rise of Civilization.* New Haven, Conn.: Yale University Press.

141. —. 1987. "The Significance of Long-Term Changes in Human Diet and Food Economy." In Harris and Ross, eds., 1987, 261–85.

142. Cohen, P., M. Miyazaki, N. D. Socci, et al. 2002. "Role for Stearoyl-CoA Desaturase-l in Leptin-Mediated Weight Loss." *Science.* July 12; 297(5579):240–43.

143. Cohn, V. 1981. "linking of Heart Disease to High-Cholesterol Diet Reinforced by New Data." *Washington Post.* Jan. 8; A14.

144. —. 1980. "A Passion to Keep Fit: 100 Million Americans Exercising." *Washington Post.* Aug. 31; AI.

145. Cook, C. H., and I. T. Whittemore. 1893. *Among the Pimas, or, The Mission to the Pima and Maricopa Indians.* Albany, N.Y.: Ladies' Union Mission School Association.

146. Cooperative Study of Lipoproteins and Atherosclerosis. 1956. "Evaluation of Serum Lipoprotein and Cholesterol Measurements as Predictors of Clinical Complications of Atherosclerosis: Report of a

Cooperative Study of Lipoproteins and Atherosclerosis." *Circulation.* Oct.; 14(4, pt. 2):691–742.

147. Cordain, L., J. B. Miller, S. B. Eaton, N. Mann, S. H. Holt, and J. D. Speth. 2000. "Plant Animal Subsistence Ratios and Macronutrient Energy Estimations in Worldwide Hunter-Gatherer Diets." *American Journal of* Clinical *Nutrition.* March; 71(3):682–92.

148. Coulston, A. M., and G. M. Reaven. 1997. "Much Ado About (Almost) Nothing." *Diabetes Care.* March; 20(3):241–43.

149. Cowie, C. C., K. F. Rust, D. D. Byrd-Holt, et al. 2006. "Prevalence of Diabetes and Impaired Fasting Glucose in Adults in the U.S. Population: National Health and Nutrition Examination Survey, 1999–2002." *Diabetes Care.* June; 29(6):1263–68.

150. Crapo, P. A., G. Reaven, and J. Olefsky. 1977. "Postprandial Plasma-Glucose and –Insulin Responses to Different Complex Carbohydrates." *Diabetes. 26(12):1178–83.*

151. Critser, G. 2003. *Fat Land: How Americans Became the Fattest People in the World.* New York: Houghton Mifflin.

152. Croftan. A. C. 1906. "The Dietetics of Obesity." *JAMA.* July–Dec.; 47: 820–23.

153. Cunningham, B. 1996. W. H. 'Bold' Emory's Notes of a Military Reconnaissance: A Survey of Arizona's Gila River, 1846." *Smoke Signal.* Fall; 66:106–15.

154. Curtain, L. S. 1949. *By the Prophet of the Earth: Ethtnobotany of the Pima.* Tucson: University of Arizona Press.

155. Dabelea, D., W. C. Knowler, and D. J. Pettitt. 2000. "Effect of Diabetes in Pregnancy on Offspring: Follow-Up Research in the Pima Indians." *Journal of Maternal and Fetal Medicine.* Jan.–Feb.; 9(1):83–88.

156. Danforth, E., Jr. 1985. "Diet and Obesity." *American Journal of Clinical Nutrition.* May; 41(5 suppl.):1132–45.

157. Dansinger, M. L., J. A. Gleason, J. L. Griffith, H. P. Selker, and E. J. Schaefer. 2005. "Comparison of the Atkins, Omish, Weight Watchers. and Zone Diets for Weight Loss and Heart Disease Risk Reduction: A Randomized Trial." *JAMA.* Jan. 5; 293(1):43–53.

158. Davis, G. P., Jr. 1962. N. B. Carmony and D. F. Brown, eds. *Man and Wildlife in Arizona:*

159. The *American Exploration Period, 1824–1865.* Scottsdale, Ariz.: Arizona Game and Fish Dept.

160. Dawber, T. R. 1980. The *Framingham Study: The Epidemiology of Atherosclerotic Disease.* Cambridge, Mass.: Harvard University Press.

161. —. 1978. "Annual Discourse-Unproved Hypotheses." *New England Journal of Medicine.* Aug. 31; 299(9):452–58.

162. —. 1962. "The Epidemiology of Coronary Heart Disease—The Framingham Enquiry." **In** "Symposium on Arteriosclerosis," *Proceedings of the Royal Society of Medicine.* April; 55:265–71.

163. Day, J., M. Carruthers, A. Bailey, and D. Robinson. 1976. "Anthropometric, Physiological, and Biochemical Differences Between Urban and Rural Maasai." *Atherosclerosis.* 23(2):357–6I.

164. DeFronzo, R. A. 1997. "Insulin Resistance: A Multifaceted Syndrome Responsible for NIDDM, Obesity, Hypertension, Dyslipidaemia, and Atherosclerosis." *Netherlands Journal of Medicine.* May; 50(5):191–97.

165. —. 1992. "Insulin Resistance, Hyperinsulinemia, and Coronary Artery Disease: A Complex Metabolic Web." *Journal of Cardiovascular Pharmacology.* 20 (II suppl.): SI-16.

166. DeFronzo, R. A., J. D. Tobin, and R. Andres. 1979. "Glucose Clamp Technique: A Method for Quantifying Insulin Secretion and Resistance." *American Journal of Physiology.* Sept.; 237(3):E214–23.

167. Deshaies, Y., A. Dagnault, A. Boivin, and D. Richard. 1994. "Tissue- and Gender-Specific Modulation of Lipoprotein Lipase in Intact and Gonadectomised Rats Treated with D1Fenfluramine." *International Journal of Obesity and Related Metabolic Disorders.* June; 18(6):405–11.

168. Diamond, J. 2003. "The Double Puzzle of Diabetes." *Nature.* June 5; 423(6940): 599–602.

169. —. 1987. "The Worst Mistake in the History of the Human Race." *Discover.* May; 64–66.

170. Dickens, F., P. J. Randle, and W. J. Whelan, eds. 1968. *Carbohydrate Metabolism and Its*

171. *Disorders.* 2 vols. New York: Academic Press.

172. Dietary Guidelines Advisory Committee. 2005. "2005 Dietary Guidelines Advisory Committee Report." U.S. Department of Health and Human Services and U.S. Department of Agriculture. Online at http://www.health.gov/DietaryGuidelines/dga2005/ report/.

173. Dills, W. L., Jr. 1983. "Protein Fructosylation: Fructose and the Maillard Reaction." *Ameri*

174. *can journal of Clinical Nutrition*. Nov.; 58(5 suPPl.):779S–787S.

175. Dobyns, H. F. 1989. *The Pima-Maricopa*. New York: Chelsea House.

176. —. 1978. "Who Killed the Gila." *Journal of Arizona History*. 19(1):17–30.

177. Doll, R., and B. Armstrong. 1981. "Cancer." In Trowell and Burkitt, eds., 1981, 93–112. Doll, R., and R. Peto. 1981. "The Causes of Cancer. Quantitative Estimates of Avoidable Risks of Cancer in the United States Today." *Journal of the National Cancer Institute*. June; 66(6):1191–308.

178. Donahoo, W. T., D. R. Jensen, T. Y. Shepard, and R. H. Eckel. 2000. "Seasonal Variation in Lipoprotein Lipase and Plasma Lipids in Physically Active, Normal Weight Humans." *Journal of* Clinical *Endocrinology & Metabolism*. Sept.; 85(9):3065–68.

179. Donnelly, R., A. M. Emslie-Smith, I. D. Gardner, and A. D. Morris. 2000. "ABC of Arterial and Venous Disease: Vascular Complications of Diabetes." *British journal of Medicine*. April 15; 320(7241):1062–66.

180. Dreon, D. M., H. A. Fernstrom, H. Campos, P. Blanche, P. T. Williams, and R. M. Krauss. 1998. "Change in Dietary Saturated Fat Intake Is Correlated with Change in Mass of Large Low-Density-Lipoprotein Particles in Men." *American Journal of Clinical Nutrition*. May; 67(5):828–36.

181. Du Bois, E. F. 1936. *Basal Metabolism in Health and Disease*. 2nd edition. Philadelphia: Lea & Febiger.

182. Duff, G. L., and G. C. McMillan. 1949. "Effect of Alloxan Diabetes on Experimental Cholesterol Atherosclerosis in the Rabbit." *Journal of Experimental Medicine*. 89(6):611–30.

183. Dwyer, J., and D. Lu. 1993. "Popular Diets for Weight Loss: From Nutritionally Hazardous to Healthful." In Stunkard and Wadden, eds., 1993, 231–52.

184. Dyer, A. R., J. Stamler, O. Paul, et al. 1981. "Serum Cholesterol and Risk of Death from Cancer and Other Causes in Three Chicago Epidemiological Studies." *Journal of Chronic Diseases*. 34(6):249–60.

185. Eades, M. R., and M. D. Eades. 1996. *Protein Power*. New York: Bantam Books. Easterbrook, G. 1997. "Forgotten Benefactor of Humanity." *Atlantic Monthly*. Jan.; 279(1):75–82.

186. Eaton, S. B., and M. Konner. 1985. "Paleolithic Nutrition: A Consideration of Its Nature and Current Implications." *New England Journal of Medicine.* Jan. 31; 312(5):283–89.

187. Eaton, S. B., M. Shostak, and M. Konner. 1988. *The Paleolithic Prescription.* New York: Harper & Row.

188. Eccleston, R. 1950. *Overland to California on the Southwestern Trail: Diary of Robert Eccleston.* Berkeley: University of California Press.

189. Eckel, R. H. 2003. "Obesity: A Disease or a Physiological Adaptation for Survival." In Eckel, ed., 2003, 3–30.

190. Eckel, R. H., ed. 2003. *Obesity. Mechanisms and Clinical Management.* New York: Lippincott Williams & Wilkins.

191. Erlichman, J., A. L. Kerbey, and W. P. James. 2002. "Physical Activity and Its Impact on Health Outcomes. Paper 2, Prevention of Unhealthy Weight Gain and Obesity by Physical Activity: An Analysis of the Evidence." *Obesity Review.* Nov.; 3(4):273–87.

192. Ezell, P. H. 1961. "The Hispanic Acculturation of the Gila River Pimas." American Anthropological Association Memoir 90. Oct.; 63(5 pt. 2).

193. Farquhar, J. W., A. Frank, R. C. Gross, and G. M. Reaven. 1966. "Glucose, Insulin, and Triglyceride Responses to High and Low Carbohydrate Diets in Man." *Journal of Clinical Investigation.* Oct.; 45(10):1648–56.

194. Farris, W., S. Mansourian, Y. Chang, et al. 2003. "Insulin-Degrading Enzyme Regulates the Levels of Insulin, Amyloid Beta.Protein, and the Beta-Amyloid Precursor Protein Intracellular Domain in Vivo." *Proceedings of the National Academy of Sciences.* April 1; 100(7):4162–67.

195. Farris, W., S. Mansourian, M. A. Leissring, et al. 2004. "Partial Loss-of-Function Mutations in Insulin-Degrading Enzyme That Induce Diabetes Also Impair Degradation of Amyloid Beta.Protein." *American Journal of Pathology.* April; 164(4):1425–34.

196. Feener, E. P., and V. J. Dzau. 2005. "Pathogenesis of Cardiovascular Disease in Diabetes." In Kahn et al., eds., 2005, 867–84.

197. Feinleib, M.. 1981. "On a Possible Inverse Relationship Between Serum Cholesterol and Cancer Mortality." *American Journal of Epidemiology.* July; 114(1):5–10.

198. Filozof, C., M. C. Fernandez Pinilla, and A. Fernandez-Cruz. 2004. "Smoking Cessation and Weight Gain." *Obesity Reviews.* May; 5(2):95–103.

199. Flatt, J. P. 1978. *The Composition of Energy Expenditure and Its Influence on Energy Balance.* In Bray, ed., 1978, 211–28.

200. Fogelholm, M., and K. Kukkonen-Harjula. 2000. "Does Physical Activity Prevent Weight Gain—A Systematic Review." *Obesity Reviews.* Oct.; 1(2):95-111.

201. Food and Nutrition Board, National Research Council [NRC]. 1980. *Toward Healthful Diets.* Pamphlet. Washington, D.C.: National Academy of Sciences.

202. Ford, E. S., A. H. Mokdad, W. H. Giles, and D. W. Brown. 2003. "The Metabolic Syndrome and Antioxidant Concentrations: Findings from the Third National Health and Nutrition Examination Survey." *Diabetes.* Sept.; 52(9):2346–52.

203. Foster, G. D., H. R. Wyatt, J. O. Hill, et aI. 2003. "A Randomized Trial of a Low

204. Carbohydrate Diet for Obesity." *New England Journal of Medicine.* 22; 348(21): 2082–90.

205. Fouche, F. P. 1923. "Freedom of Negro Races from Cancer." *British Medical Journal.* June 30:1116.

206. Fox, C. S., M. J. Pencina, J. B. Meigs, R. S. Vasan, Y. S. Levitzky, and R. B. D'Agostino, Sr. 2006. "Trends in the Incidence of Type 2 Diabetes Mellitus from the 1970s to the 1990s: The Framingham Heart Study." *Circulation.* June 27; 113(25):2914–18.

207. Franz, M. J., J. P. Bantle, C. A. Beebe, et al. 2003. "American Diabetes Association: Evidence-Based Nutrition Principles and Recommendations for the Treatment and Prevention of Diabetes and Related Complications." *Diabetes Care.* Jan.; 26 (suppl. 1):S51–61.

208. Fraser, G. E., J. T. Anderson, N. Foster, R. Goldberg, D. Jacobs, and H. Blackburn. 1983. "The Effect of Alcohol on Serum High Density Lipoprotein (HDL): A Controlled Experiment." *Atherosclerosis.* March; 46(3):275–86.

209. Fredrickson, D. S., R. I. Levy, and R. S. Lees. 1967a. "Fat Transport in Lipoproteins: An Integrated Approach to Mechanisms and Disorders." *New England Journal of Medicine.* Feb. 2; 276(5):273–81.

210. —. 1967b. "Fat Transport in Lipoproteins: An Integrated Approach to Mechanisms and Disorders. *New England Journal of Medicine.* Jan. 26; 276(4):215–25.

211. —. 1967c. "Fat Transport in Lipoproteins: An Integrated Approach to Mechanisms and Disorders. i*n New England Journal of Medicine.* Jan. 19; 276(3):148–56.

212. —. 1967d. "Fat Transport in Lipoproteins: An Integrated Approach to Mechanisms and Disorders. *n New England Journal of Medicine.* Jan. 12; 276(2):94–103.

213. —. 1967e. "Fat Transport in Lipoproteins: An Integrated Approach to Mechanisms and Disorders: *New England Journal of Medicine.* Jan. 5; 276(1):34–42.

214. *Circulation.* May; 17(5):852–61.

215. Friedman, J. M. 2004. "Modem Science Versus the Stigma of Obesity: *Nature Medicine.* June; 10(6):563–69.

216. —. 2003. "A War on Obesity, Not the Obese: *Science.* Feb. 7; 299(5608):856–58. Friedman, M. 1969. *Pathogenesis of Coronary Artery Disease.* New York: McGraw-Hill. Friedman, M. I., and E. M. Stricker. 1976. "The Physiological Psychology of Hunger: A Physiological Perspective." *Psychological Review.* Nov.; 83(6):409–31.

217. Friend, B., 1. Page, and R. Marston. 1979. "Food Consumption Patterns, U.S.A.: 1909–13 to 1976." In *Nutrition, Lipids, and Coronary Heart Disease: A Global View,* ed. R. I. Levy, B. M. Rifkind, B. H. Dennis, and N. Ernst. New York: Raven Press, 489–522.

218. Fritz, I. B. 1961. "Factors Influencing the Rates of Long-Chain Fatty Acid Oxidation and Synthesis in Mammalian Systems." *Physiological Reviews.* Jan.; 41:52–129.

219. Furnas, C. C., and S. M. Furnas. 1937. *Man, Bread, and Destiny: The Story of Man and His Food.* New York: New Home Library.

220. Gabbay, K. H., K. Hasty, J. L. Breslow, R. C. Ellison, H. F. Bunn, and P. M. Gallop. 1977. "Glycosylated Hemoglobins and Long-Term Blood Glucose Control in Diabetes Mellitus: *Journal of Clinical Endocrinology* III *Metabolism.* May; 44(5):859–64.

221. Gale, E. A. 2002. "The Rise of Childhood Type I Diabetes in the 20th Century." *Diabetes.*

222. Dec.; 51(12):3353–61.

223. Garcia-Palmieri, M. R., P. D. Sorlie, R. Costas, Jr., and R. J. Havlik. 1981. "An Apparent

224. —. Inverse Relationship Between Serum Cholesterol and Cancer Mortality in Puerto Rico." *American Journal of Epidemiology.* July; 114(1):29–40.

225. Garcia-Palmieri, M. R., P. Sorlie, J. Tillotson, R. Costas, Jr., E. Cordero, and M. Rodriguez. 1980. "Relationship of Dietary Intake to Subsequent Coronary Heart Disease Incidence: The Puerto Rico Heart Health Program." *American Journal of Clinical Nutrition.* Aug.; 33(8):1818–27.

226. Omish, and LEARN Diets for Change in Weight and Related Risk Factors Among Overweight Premenopausal Women: The A TO Z Weight Loss Study: A Randomized Trial." *JAMA.* March 7; 297(9):969–77.

227. Garrow, J. S. 1981. *Treat Obesity Seriously.* New York: Churchill Livingstone.

228. —. 1978. *Energy Balance and Obesity in Man.* New York: Elsevier/ North-Holland Biomedical Press.

229. Gerrior, S., and L. Bente. 2001. *Nutrient Content of the U.S. Food Supply, 1909–1997.* U.S. Department of Agriculture Center for Nutrition Policy and Promotion Home Economics Research Report No. 54.

230. Gershoff, S. N. 2001. "Jean Mayer 1920–1993'" *Journal of Nutrition.* June; 131(6):1651–54.

231. Giovannucci, E. 2001. "Insulin, Insulin-Like Growth Factors, and Colon Cancer: A Review of the Evidence." *Journal of Nutrition.* Nov.; 131(II suppl.):3109S–20S.

232. Giovannucci, E., E. B. Rimm, M. J. Stampfer, G. A. Colditz, A. Ascherio, and W. C. Willett. 1994. "Intake of Fat, Meat, and Fiber in Relation to Risk of Colon Cancer in Men." *Cancer Research.* May I; 54(9):2390–97.

233. Giugliano, D., A. Ceriello, and G. Paolisso. 1996. "Oxidative Stress and Diabetic Vascular Complications." *Diabetes Care.* March; 19(3):257–67.

234. Gladwell, M. 1998. "The Pima Paradox." *New Yorker.* Feb. 2. Online at http://www.gladwell.com/1998/1998_02_02_a_pima.htm.

235. Glinsmann, W. H., H. Irausquin, and Y. K. Park. 1986. "Report from FDA's Sugars Task

236. Force, 1986: Evaluation of Health Aspects of Sugars Contained in Carbohydrate Sweeteners." *Journal of Nutrition*. Nov.; n6(II suppl.):sl-s216.

237. Glueck, C. J. 1979. Appraisal of Dietary Fat as a Causative Factor in Atherogenesis." *American Journal of Clinical Nutrition*. Dec.; 32(12 suppl.):2637–43.

238. Gofman, J. W. 1958. "Diet in the Prevention and Treatment of Myocardial Infarction," *American Journal of Cardiology*. Feb.; 1(2):271–83.

239. Gofman, J. W., and F. P. Lindgren. 1950. "The Role of Lipids and Lipoproteins in Atherosclerosis." *Science*. Feb. 17; m(2877):166–86.

240. Gofman, J. W., A. V. Nichols. and E. V. Dobbin. 1958. *Dietary Prevention and Treatment of Heart Disease*. New York: Putnam.

241. Gofman, J. W., and W. Young. 1963. "The Filtration Concept of Atherosclerosis and Serum Lipids in the Diagnosis of Atherosclerosis." In Sandler and Bourne, eds., 1963, 197–23°.

242. Gofman, J. W., W. Young, and R. Tandy. 1966. "Ischemic Heart Disease, Atherosclerosis, and Longevity." *Circulation*. Oct.; 34(4):679–97.

243. Golay, A., and E. Bobbioni. 1997. "The Role of Dietary Fat in Obesity." *International Jour*nal *of Obesity and Related Metabolic Disorders*. June; 21(3 suppl.):S2–11.

244. Goldberg, C. 2006. "Weight Risk on the Rise for Infants." *Boston Globe*. Aug. 10; AI. Goldberg, L., D. L. Elliot, R. W. Schutz, and F. E. Kloster. 1984. "Changes in Lipid and Lipoprotein Levels After Weight Training." *JAMA*. July 27; 252(4):504–6.

245. Goldblatt, P. B., M.E. Moore, and A. J. Stunkard. 1965. "Social Factors in Obesity." *JAMA*. June 21; 192:1039–44.

246. Goldman, R. F., M. F. Haisman, G. Bynum, E. S. Horton, and E. A. Sims. 1976. "Experimental Obesity in Man: Metabolic Rate in Relation to Dietary Intake." In Bray, ed., 1976b, 165–86.

247. Gordon, E. S. 1970. "Metabolic Aspects of Obesity." *Advances in Metabolic Disorders*. 4:229–96.

248. Gordon, T. 1988. "The Diet-Heart Idea: Outline of a History." *American Journal of Epidemiology*. Feb.; 127(2):220–25.

249. Gordon, T., W. P. Castelli, M. C. Hjortland, W. B. Kannel, and T. R. Dawber. 1977. "High Density Lipoprotein as a Protective Factor Against Coronary Heart Disease: The Framingham Study." *American Journal of Medicine*. May; 62(5):707–14.

250. Gracey, M., N. Kretchmer, and E. Rossi, eds. 1991. *Sugars in Nutrition.* New York: Raven Press.

251. Grande, F., J. T. Anderson, and A. Keys. 1958. "Changes of Basal Metabolic Rate in Man in Semistarvation and Refeeding: *Journal of Applied Physiology.* March; 12(2):230–38.

252. Greene, R. 1970. *Human Hormones.* New York: McGraw-Hill.

253. Greenwood, M. R. 1985. "Normal and Abnormal Growth and Maintenance of Adipose Tissue." In Hirsch and Van ltallie, eds., 1985, 20–25.

254. Greenwood, M. R., M. Cleary, L. Steingrimsdottir, and J. R. Vaselli. 1981. "Adipose Tissue Metabolism and Genetic Obesity." In Bjorntorp, Cairella, and Howard, eds., 1981, 75–79.

255. Grey, N., and D. M. Kipnis. 1971. "Effect of Diet Composition on the Hyperinsulinemia of Obesity." *New England Journal of Medicine.* Oct. 7; 285(15):827–31.

256. Griffin, J. S. 1943. A *Doctor Comes to California: The Diary of John S. Griffin, Assistant Surgeon with Kearny's Dragoons,* 1846–1847. San Francisco: California Historical Society.

257. Grossman, H. 2003. "Does Diabetes Protect or Provoke Alzheimer's Disease? Insights into the Pathobiology and Future Treatment of Alzheimer's Disease." *CNS Spectrum.* Nov.; 8(II):815–23.

258. Grundy, S. M. 1994. "Influence of Stearic Acid on Cholesterol Metabolism Relative to Other Long-Chain Fatty Acids." *American Journal of Clinical Nutrition.* Dec.; 60(6 suppl.):986S–90S.

259. Grundy, S. M., H. B. Brewer, Jr., J. I. Cleeman, S. C. Smith, Jr., and C. Lenfant. 2004. "Definition of Metabolic Syndrome: Report of the National Heart, Lung, and Blood Institute/American Heart Association Conference on Scientific Issues Related to Definition." *Circulation.* Jan. 27; 109(3):433–38.

260. Grundy, S. M., B. Hansen, S. C. Smith, Jr., J. I. Cleeman, and R. A. Kahn. 2004. "Clinical Management of Metabolic Syndrome: Report of the American Heart Association/ National Heart, Lung, and Blood Institute/American Diabetes Association Conference on Scientific Issues Related to Management." *Circulation.* Feb. 3; 109(4):551–56.

261. Guery, P., and M. C. Secretin. 1991. "Sugars and Non-Nutritive Sweeteners." In Gracey, Kretchmer, and Rossi, eds., 1991, 33–54.

262. Gwinup, G. 1974. "Effects of Diet and Exercise in the Treatment of Obesity." In Bray and Bethune, eds., 1974, 93–102.

263. Hammond, M. G., and W. R. Fisher. 1971. "The Characterization of a Discrete Series of Low Density Lipoproteins in the Disease, Hyper-Pre-Beta-Lipoproteinemia: Implications Relating to the Structure of Plasma Lipoproteins." *Journal of* Biological *Chemistry*. Sept. 10; 246(17):5454–65.

264. Han, P. W., and L W. Frohman. 1970. "Hyperinsulinemia in Tube-Fed Hypophysectomized Rats Bearing Hypothalamic Lesions." *American Journal of Physiology*. Dec.; 219(6): 1632–36.

265. Harper. A. E. 1996. "Dietary Guidelines in Perspective." *Journal of Nutrition*. April; 126(4 suppl.):1042S–48S.

266. Havel, P. J. 2005. "Dietary Fructose: Implications for Dysregulation of Energy Homeostasis and Lipid/Carbohydrate Metabolism: *Nutrition Review*. May; 63(5):133–57.

267. Hedrick. C. C.. S. R. Thorpe. M. X. Fu. et al. 2000. "Glycation Impairs High Density lipoprotein Function: *Diabetologia*. March; 43(3):312–20.

268. Heini. A. F., and R. L. Weinsier. 1997. "Divergent Trends in Obesity and Fat Intake Patterns: The American Paradox: *American Journal of Medicine*. March; 102(3):259–64.

269. Hesse. F. G. 1959. "A Dietary Study of the Pima Indian." *American Journal of Clinical Nutrition*. Sept.–Oct.; 7:532–37.

270. Hesser, L. 2006. The *Man Who Fed the World: Nobel Peace Prize Laureate Norman Borlaug and His Battle* to *End World Hunger*. Dallas: Durban House.

271. Higgins, H. L. 1916. "The Rapidity with Which Alcohol and Some Sugars May Serve as Nutriment." *American Journal of Physiology*. Aug.; 41(2):258–265.

272. Higginson, J. 1997. "From Geographical Pathology to Environmental Carcinogenesis: A Historical Reminiscence." *Cancer Letters*. *117:133–42*.

273. Hirsch, J. 1985. "Dietary Treatment" In Hirsch and Van ltallie, eds., 1985, 192–95.

274. —. 1978. "Obesity: A Perspective." In Bray, ed., 1978, 1–5.

275. Hirsch, J., and T. B. Van ltallie, eds. 1985. *Recent Advances in Obesity Research: IV*. London: John Libbey.

276. Hollenbeck, C. 1993. "Dietary Fructose Effects on Lipoprotein Metabolism and Risk for Coronary Disease." *American Journal of Clinical Nutrition.* Nov.; 58(5 suppl.): 800s–809s.

277. Holzenberger, M., J. Dupont, B. Ducos. et al. 2003. "IGF-l Receptor Regulates Life span and Resistance to Oxidative Stress in Mice." *Nature.* Jan. 9; 421(6919): 182–87.

278. Horton, E. S., E. Danforth, Jr.. and E. A. Sims. 1974. "Endocrine and Metabolic Alterations Associated with Overfeeding and Obesity in Man." In Burland, Samuel, and Yudkin. eds., 1974, 229–51.

279. Howard, B. V., J. E. Manson, M. L. Stefanick, et al. 2006. "Low-Fat Dietary Pattern and Weight Change over 7 Years: The Women's Health Initiative Dietary Modification Trial." *JAMA.* Jan. 4; 295(1):39–49.

280. Howard. B. V., L. Van Horn. J. Hsia. et al. 2006. "Low-Fat Dietary Pattern and Risk of Cardiovascular Disease: The Women's Health Initiative Randomized Controlled Dietary Modification Trial: *JAMA.* Feb. 8; 295(6):655–66.

281. Howell. W. H., D. J. McNamara, M. A. Tosca. B. T. Smith. and J. A. Gaines. 1997. "Plasma Lipid and Lipoprotein Responses to Dietary Fat and Cholesterol: A Meta-Analysis."*American Journal of Clinical Nutrition.* June; 65(6):1747–64.

282. Hrdlicka, A. 1908. *Physiological and Medical Observations Among the Indians of Southwestem United States and Northern Mexico.* Washington D.C.: U.S. Government Printing Office.

283. —. 1906. "Notes on the Pima of Arizona: *American Anthropologist.* Jan.–March; 8(1):39–46.

284. Hulley, S. B., J. M. Walsh, and T. B. Newman. 1992. "Health Policy on Blood Cholesterol: Time to Change Directions." *Circulation.* Sept.; 86(3):1026–29.

285. Hunink, M. G., L. Goldman, A. N. Tosteson, et al. 1997. "The Recent Decline in Mortality from Coronary Heart Disease, 1980–1990: The Effect of Secular Trends in Risk Factors and Treatment." *JAMA.* Feb. 19; 277(7):535–42.

286. Hustvedt, B. A, and A Lovo. 1972. "Correlation Between Hyperinsulinemia and Hyperphagia in Rats with Ventromedial Hypothalamic Lesions." *Acta Physiologica Scandinavica.* Jan.; 84(1):29–33.

287. Hwang, I. S., B. B. Hoffman, and G. M. Reaven. 1987. "Fructose-Induced Insulin Resistance and Hypertension in Rats." *Hypertension.* Nov.; 10(5):512–16.

288. Institute of Medicine [10M] of the National Academies. 2002. *Dietary Reference Intakes: Energy, Carbohydrate, Fiber, Fat, Fatty Acids, Cholesterol, Protein, and Amino Acids.* Washington, D.C.: National Academies Press.

289. —. 1995. *Weighing the Options: Criteria for Evaluating Weight-Management Programs.* Washington, D.C.: National Academy Press.

290. Jackson, Y. M. 1994. "Diet. Culture, and Diabetes." In Joe and Young. eds., 1994.381–406.

291. Jacobs, D., H. Blackburn, M. Higgins, et al. 1992. "Report of the Conference on Low Blood Cholesterol: Mortality Associations." *Circulation.* Sept.; 86(3):1046–60.

292. Jacobson, M. 1978. "The Deadly White Powder." *Mother Jones.* July; 12–20.

293. Janssen, G. M., C. J. Graef, and W. H. Saris. 1989. "Food Intake and Body Composition in Novice Athletes During a Training Period to Run a Marathon." *International Journal of Sports Medicine.* May; 10(1 suppl.):SI7–21.

294. Jeanrenaud, B. 1979. "Insulin and Obesity." *Diabetologia.* Sept.; 17(3):133–38.

295. Jeffery, R. W., W. L. Hellerstedt, S. A. French, and J. E. Baxter. 1995. "A Randomized Trial of Counseling for Fat Restriction Versus Calorie Restriction in the Treatment of Obesity." *International Journal of Obesity and Related Metabolic Disorders.* Feb.; 19(2):132–37.

296. Jenkins, D. J., T. M. Wolever, R. H. Taylor, et al. 1981. "Glycemic Index of Foods: A Physiological Basis for Carbohydrate Exchange." *American Journal of Clinical Nutrition.* March; 34(3):362–66.

297. Joslin Diabetes Center. 2003. Press Release: "Study Shows It May Someday Be Possible to Stay Slim, Avoid Type 2 Diabetes and Live Longer—While Eating What You Want." Jan. 23.

298. Joslin, E. P. 1940. "The Universality of Diabetes: A Survey of Diabetes Morbidity in Arizona." *JAMA.* Oct.–Dec.; 115:2033–38.

299. Joslin, E. P., H. F. Root, P. White, and A. Marble, eds. 1959. The *Treatment of Diabetes Mellitus.* 10th edition. Philadelphia: Lea & Febiger.

300. Kaaks, R., and A. Lukanova. 2001. "Energy Balance and Cancer: The Role of Insulin and Insulin-Like Growth Factor-I." *Proceedings of the Nutrition Society.* Feb.; 60(1):91–106.

301. Kahn, C. R., and G. C. Weir, eds. 1994. *Joslin's Diabetes Mellitus.* 13th edition. Media, Pa.: Lippincott Williams & Wilkins.

302. Kahn, C. R., G. C. Weir, G. L. King, A. M. Jacobson, A. C. Moses, and R. J. Smith, eds. 2005. *Joslin's Diabetes Mellitus.* 14th edition. New York: Lippincott Williams & Wilkins.

303. Kahn, H. A., J. H. Medalie, H. N. Neufeld, E. Riss, M. Balogh, and J. J. Groen. 1969. "Serum Cholesterol: Its Distribution and Association with Dietary and Other Variables in a Survey of 10,000 Men." *Israeli Journal of Medical Sciences.* Nov.–Dec.; 5(6):III7–27.

304. Kannel, W. B., W. P. Castelli, and T. Gordon. 1979. "Cholesterol in the Prediction of Atherosclerotic Disease: New Perspectives Based on the Framingham Study." *Annals of Internal Medicine.* Jan.; 90(1):85–91.

305. Kannel, W. B., W. P. Castelli, T. Gordon, and P. M. McNamara. 1971. "Serum Cholesterol, Lipoproteins, and the Risk of Coronary Heart Disease: The Framingham Study." *Annals of Internal Medicine.* Jan.; 74(1):1–12.

306. Kannel, W. B., and T. Gordon. 1968. The *Framingham Diet Study: Diet and Regulation of Serum Cholesterol.* Sect. 24 of The *Framingham Study: An Epidemiological Investigation of Cardiovascular Disease.* Bethesda. Md.: U.S. Department of Health, Education. and Welfare, Public Health Service. and National Institutes of Health.

307. Kannel, W. B., and H. E. Thomas, Jr. 1982. "Sudden Coronary Death: The Framingham Study." *Annals of the New York Academy of Sciences.* March; 382:3–21.

308. Katz, L. N., J. Stamler, and R. Pick. 1958. *Nutrition and Atherosclerosis.* Philadelphia: Lea & Febiger.

309. Kaunitz, H. 1977. "Importance of lipids in Arteriosclerosis: An Outdated Theory." In Select Committee on Nutrition and Human Needs of the United States Senate 1977c, 42–54.

310. Keesey, R. 1980. "A Set. Point Analysis of the Regulation of Body Weight." In Stunkard, ed., 1980, 144–65.

311. Kekwick, A., and G. L. Pawan. 1957. "Metabolic Study in Human Obesity with Isocaloric Diets High in Fat, Protein, or Carbohydrate." *Metabolism Clinical and Experimental.* 6(5):447–60.

312. Kennedy, E. T., S. A. Bowman, J. T. Spence, M. Freedman, and J. King. 2001. "Popular Diets: Correlation to Health, Nutrition, and Obesity." *Journal of the American Dietetic Association.* April; 101(4):411–20.

313. Kenyon, C. 2001. "A Conserved Regulatory System for Aging." *Cell.* April 20; 105(2): 165–68.

314. Kenyon, c., J. Chang, E. Gensch, A. Rudner, and R. Tabtiang. 1993. "A C. Elegans Mutant That lives Twice As Long As Wild Type." *Nature.* Dec. 2; 366(6454):461–64.

315. Kern, P. A., J. M. Ong, B. Saffari, and J. Carty. 1990. "The Effects of Weight Loss on the Activity and Expression of Adipose-Tissue lipoprotein lipase in Very Obese Humans." *New England Journal of Medicine.* April 12; 322(15):1053–59.

316. Keys A. 1994. "The Inception and Pilot Surveys." In *The Seven Countries Study. A Scientific Adventure in Cardiovascular Disease Epidemiology,* ed. D. Kromhout, A. Menotti, and H. Blackburn. Utrecht: Brouwer, 15–26.

317. —. 1980. *Seven Countries: A Multivariate Analysis of Death and Coronary Heart Disease.* Cambridge, Mass.: Harvard University Press.

318. —. 1975. "Coronary Heart Disease: The Global Picture." *Atherosclerosis.* Sept.–Oct.; 22(2):149–92.

319. —. 1971. "Sucrose in the Diet and Coronary Heart Disease." *Atherosclerosis.* Sept.–Oct.; 14(2):193–202.

320. —. ed. 1970. "Coronary Heart Disease in Seven Countries." *Circulation.* April 4; 41(4suppl.):I:1–2II.

321. —. 1966. "Arteriosclerotic Heart Disease in Roseto, Pennsylvania." *JAMA.* Jan. 10; 195(2):93–95.

322. —. 1963. "The Role of the Diet in Human Atherosclerosis and Its Complications." In Sandler and Bourne, eds., 1963, 263–301.

323. —. 1957. "Diet and the Epidemiology of Coronary Heart Disease." *JAMA.* Aug. 24; 164(17):1912–19.

324. —. 1953. "Atherosclerosis: A Problem in Newer Public Health." *Journal of Mount Sinai Hospital, New York.* July–Aug.; 20(2):118–39.

325. —. 1952. "Human Atherosclerosis and the Diet." *Circulation.* Jan.; 5(1):115–18.

326. —. 1949. "The Calorie Requirement of Adult Man." *Nutrition Abstracts and Reviews.* July; 19:1–10.

327. Keys, A., and J. T. Anderson. 1955. "The Relationship of the Diet to the Development of Atherosclerosis in Man." In *Symposium on Atherosclerosis,* pub. no. 338. Washington, D.C.: National Research Council, National Academy of Sciences, 181–97.

328. Keys, A., J. T. Anderson, F. Fidanza, M. H. Keys, and B. Swahn. 1955. "Effects of Diet on Blood Lipids in Man, Particularly Cholesterol and Lipoproteins." *Clinical Chemistry.* Feb.; 1(1):34–52.

329. Keys, A., J. T. Anderson, and F. Grande. 1957. "Prediction of Serum-Cholesterol Responses of Man to Changes in Fats in the Diet." *Lancet.* Nov. 16; 273(7003):959–66.

330. Keys, A., J. T. Anderson, O. Mickelsen, S. F. Adelson, and R. Fidanza. 1956. "Diet and Serum Cholesterol in Man: Lack of Effect of Dietary Cholesterol." *Journal of Nutrition.* May 10; 59(1):39–56.

331. Keys, A., and J. Brozek. 1953. "Body Fat in Adult Man." *Physiological Reviews.* July; 33(3):245–325.

332. Keys, A., J. Brozek, A. Henschel, O. Mickelsen, and H. L. Taylor. 1950. *The Biology of Human Starvation.* 2 vols. Minneapolis: University of Minnesota Press.

333. Keys, A., and M. Keys. 1975. *How to Eat* Well *and Stay* Well: *The Mediterranean Way.* Garden City, N.Y.: Doubleday.

334. —. 1959. *Eat* Well *and Stay* Well. Garden City, N.Y.: Doubleday.

335. Keys, A., N. Kimura, A. Kusukawa, B. Bronte, Stewart, N. Larsen, and M. H. Keys. 1958. "Lessons from Serum Cholesterol Studies in Japan, Hawaii and Los Angeles." *Annals of Internal Medicine.* Jan.; 48(1):83–94.

336. Keys, A., A. Menotti, C. Aravanis, et al. 1984. "The Seven Countries Study: 2,289 Deaths in 15 Years." *Preventive Medicine.* March; 13(2):141–54.

337. Keys, A., O. Mickelsen, E. O. Miller, and C. B. Chapman. 1950. "The Relation in Man Between Cholesterol Levels in the Diet and in the Blood." *Science.* July 21; II2(2899):79–81.

338. Kiens, B., H. Lithell, K. J. Mikines, and R. E. Richter. 1989. "Effects ofInsulin and Exercise on Muscle Lipoprotein Lipase Activity in Man and Its Relation to Insulin Action." *Journal of Clinical Investigation.* Oct.; 84(4):II24–29.

339. Kimura, K. D., H. A. Tissenbaum, Y. Liu, and G. Ruvkun. 1997. "Daf-2, an Insulin Receptor-Like Gene That Regulates Longevity and Diapause in Caenorhabditis Elegans." *Science.* Aug. 15; 277(5328):942–46.

340. Kinsell. L. W. 1969. "Dietary Composition-Weight Loss: Calories Do Count." In Wilson. ed.. 1969, 177–84.

341. Kleiber. M. 1961. The *Fire of Life: An Introduction to Animal Energetics.* New York: John Wiley.

342. Knowler, W. C., E. Barrett-Connor. S. E. Fowler. et al. 2002. [Diabetes 'Prevention Program Research Group.] "Reduction in the Incidence of Type 2 Diabetes with Lifestyle Intervention or Metformin." *New England Journal of Medicine.* Feb. 7; 346(6):393–403.

343. Koenig, R. J., C. M. Peterson, R. L. Jones, C. Saudek. M. Lehrman, and A. Cerami. 1976. "Correlation of Glucose Regulation and Hemoglobin AlC in Diabetes Mellitus." *New England Journal of Medicine.* Aug. 19; 295(8):417–20.

344. Koga, Y., R. Hashimoto, H. Adachi, M. Tsumta. H. Tashiro. and H. Toshima. 1994. "Recent Trends in Cardiovascular Disease and Risk Factors in the Seven Countries Study: Japan." In *Lessons for Science from the Seven Countries Study,* ed. H. Toshima, Y. Koga, and H. Blackburn. Tokyo: Springer-Verlag, 63–74.

345. Kolata. G. 2000a. "Health Advice: A Matter of Cause, Effect and Confusion," *New York Times.* April 25; Fl.

346. —. 2000b. "2 Fiber Studies Find No Benefit for the Colon." *New York Times.* April 20; AI.

347. —. 1987. "High-Carb Diets Questioned." *Science.* Jan. 9; 235(4785):164.

348. —. 1985. "Heart Panels Conclusions Questioned." *Science.* Jan. 4; 227(4682):40–41.

349. Koop, C. E. 1988. "Message from the Surgeon General." In U.S. Department of Health and Human Services, 1988.

350. Kraus, B. R. 1954. *Indian Health in Arizona: A Study of Health Conditions Among Central and Southern Arizona Indians.* Tucson: University of Arizona Press.

351. Krauss, R. M. 2005. "Dietary and Genetic Probes of Atherogenic Dyslipidemia." *Arteriosclerosis, Thrombosis, and Vascular Biology.* Nov.; 25(II):2265–'72.

352. Krauss, R. M., and D. J. Burke. 1982. "Identification of Multiple Subclasses of Plasma Low Density Lipoproteins in Normal Humans." *Journal of Lipid Research.* Jan.; 23(1):97–104.

353. Krauss, R. M., R. J. Deckelbaum, N. Ernst, et al. 1996. "Dietary Guidelines for Healthy American Adults: A Statement for Health Professionals from the Nutrition Committee, American Heart Association." *Circulation.* Oct. I; 94(7):1795–800.

354. Krauss, R. M., R. H. Eckel. B. Howard, et al. 2000. "AHA Dietary Guidelines, Revision 2000: A Statement for Healthcare Professionals from the Nutrition Committee of the American Heart Association." *Stroke.* Nov.; 31(II):2751–66.

355. Krebs, H. A 1981. *Reminiscences and Reflections.* Oxford: Clarendon Press, 1971. "How the Whole Becomes More Than the Sum of the Parts." *Perspectives in Biology and Medicine.* Spring; 14(3):448–57.

356. —. 1967. "The Making of a Scientist." *Nature.* Sept. 30; 215(5109):1441–45.

357. —. 1960. "The Cause of the Specific Dynamic Action of Food Stuffs." *Arzneimittelforschung.* May; 10:369–73.

358. Kushi, L. H., T. Byers, C. Doyle, et al. 2006. [American Cancer Society 2006 Nutrition and Physical Activity Guidelines Advisory Committee.] "American Cancer Society Guidelines on Nutrition and Physical Activity for Cancer Prevention: Reducing the Risk of Cancer with Healthy Food Choices and Physical Activity." *CA: A Cancer Journal for Clinicians.* Sept.–Oct.; 56(5):254–81.

359. Kushi, L. H., R. A. Lew, F. J. Stare, et al. 1985. "Diet and 20-Year Mortality from Coronary Heart Disease: The Ireland-Boston Diet-Heart Study: *New England Journal of Medicine.* March 28; 312(13):811–18.

360. Kuulasmaa, K., H. Tunstall-Pedoe, A Dobson, et a!. 2000. "Estimation of Contribution of Changes in Classic Risk Factors to Trends in Coronary-Event Rates Across the WHO MONICA Project Populations: *Lancet.* Feb. 26; 355(9205):675–87.

361. Landsberg, L. 2001. "Insulin-Mediated Sympathetic Stimulation: Role in the Pathogenesis of Obesity-Related Hypertension (or, How Insulin Affects Blood Pressure, and Why)." *Journal of Hypertension.* March; 19(3, pt. 2):523–28.

362. Lane. W. A. 1929. The *Prevention of the Diseases Peculiar to Civilization*. London: Faber & Faber.

363. LaRosa, J. C., A. Gordon, R. Muesing. and D. R. Rosing. 1980. "Effects of High-Protein. Low-Carbohydrate Dieting on Plasma Lipoproteins and Body Weight." *Journal of the American Dietetic Association*. Sept.; 77(3):264–70.

364. LaRosa. J. C.. D. Hunninghake, D. Bush. et al. 1990. "The Cholesterol Facts: A Summary of the Evidence Relating Dietary Fats. Serum Cholesterol. and Coronary Heart Disease: A Joint Statement by the American Heart Association and the National Heart, Lung, and Blood Institute, the Task Force on Cholesterol Issues, American Heart Association." *Circulation*. May; 81(5):1721–33.

365. Laurell, S. 1956. "Plasma Free Fatty Acids in Diabetic Acidosis and Starvation." *Scandinavian journal of Clinical and Laboratory Investigation. 8(1):81–82.*

366. Leary, T. 1935. "Atherosclerosis: The Important Form of Arteriosclerosis. a Metabolic Disease." *JAMA*. Aug. 17; 105(7):475–81.

367. Lee. R. B. 1968. "What Hunters Do for a Living, or, How to Make Out on Scarce Resources." In Lee and DeVore, eds.. 1968. 30–48.

368. Lee, R. B., and I. DeVore. 1968. "Problems in the Study of Hunters and Gatherers." In Lee and DeVore, eds., 1968. 3–12.

369. Lee, R. B., and I. DeVore, eds. 1968. *Man the Hunter*. New York: Aldine Publishing.

370. Lees. R. S.. and D. E. Wilson. 1971. "The Treatment of Hyperlipidemia." *New England Journal of Medicine*. Jan. 28; 284(4):186–95.

371. Leibel. R. L.. M. Rosenbaum, and J. Hirsch. 1995. "Changes in Energy Expenditure Resulting from Altered Body Weight." *New England Journal of Medicine*. March 9; 332(10):621–28.

372. Leith, W. 1961. "Experiences with the Pennington Diet in the Management of Obesity." *Canadian Medical Association Journal*. June 24; 84:1411–14.

373. Le Magnen, J. 2001. "My Scientific Life: 40 Years at the College de France." *Neuroscience & Biobehavioral Reviews*. July; 25(5):375–94.

374. —. 1988. "Lipogenesis, Lipolysis and Feeding Rhythms." *Annals of Endocrinology (Paris). 49(2):98–104.*

375. —. 1985. *Hunger*. Cambridge: Cambridge University Press.

376. LeRoith, D. 2004. "Blast from the Past-Insulin Does It Again'" *Journal of Clinical Endocrinology & Metabolism.* July; 89(7):3103–4.

377. LeRoith, D., R. Baserga, L Helman, and C. T. Roberts, Jr. 1995. "Insulin-Like Growth Factors and Cancer." *Annals of Internal Medicine.* Jan. I; 122(1):54–59.

378. LeRoith, D., and C. T. Roberts, Jr. 2003. "The Insulin-Like Growth Factor System and Cancer." *Cancer Letters.* June 10; 195(2):127–37.

379. Levenstein, H. 1999. "The Perils of Abundance: Food, Health, and Morality in American History." In *A Culinary History of Food,* ed. J. L. Flandrin, M. Montanari, and A. Sonnenfeld. New York: Columbia University Press, 516–29.

380. —. 1993. *Paradox of Plenty. A Social History of Eating in Modern America.* New York: Oxford University Press.

381. Levine, J. A., N. L. Eberhardt, and M. D. Jensen. 1999. "Role of Nonexercise Activity Thermogenesis in Resistance to Fat Gain in Humans." *Science.* Jan. 8; 283(5399):212–14.

382. Levy, R. I., and N. Ernst. 1976. "Diet, Hyperlipidemia, and Atherosclerosis." In Goodhart and Shils, eds., 1973, 895–918.

383. Levy, R. I., R. S. Lees, and D. S. Fredrickson. 1966. "The Nature of Pre Beta (Very Low Density) Lipoproteins." *Journal of Clinical Investigation.* Jan.; 45(1):63–77.

384. Lieb, C. W., and E. Tolstoi. 1929. "Effect of an Exclusive Meat Diet on Chemical Constituents of the Blood." *Proceedings of the Society for Experimental Biology and Medicine.* Jan.; 26(4):324–25.

385. Lin, K., J. B. Dorman, A. Rodan, and C. Kenyon. 1997. "Daf-16: An HNF-3/Forkhead Family Member That Can Function to Double the Life-Span of Caenorhabditis Elegans." *Science.* Nov. 14; 278(5341):1319–22.

386. Lin, S. J., P. A. Defossez, and L. Guarente. 2000. "Requirement of NAD and SIR2 for Life-Span Extension by Calorie Restriction in Saccharomyces Cerevisiae." *Science.* Sept. 22; 289(5487):2126–28.

387. Lindner, L. 2001. "When Good Carbs Turn Bad: Fine-Tuning the Carbohydrate-to-Fat Ratio May Reduce Heart Risks for Those with 'Syndome X.'" *n Washington Post.* June 19; T09.

388. Lipid Research Clinics [LRC] Program. 1984a. "The lipid Research Clinics Coronary Primary Prevention Trial Results. I. Reduction

in Incidence of Coronary Heart Disease." *JAMA.* Jan. 20; 251(3):351–64.

389. —. 1984b. "The lipid Research Clinics Coronary Primary Prevention Trial Results. II. The Relationship of Reduction in Incidence of Coronary Heart Disease to Cholesterol Lowering." *JAMA.* Jan. 20; 251(3):365–74.

390. —. 1979. "The Coronary Primary Prevention Trial: Design and Implementation."*Journal of Chronic Diseases. 32(9–10):609–31.*

391. Lithell, H. 1987. "Site Differences in lipoprotein Lipase Activity." In Berry et al., eds., 1987,77–81.

392. Lorgeril, M. de, P. Salen, J. L. Martin, I. Monjaud, J. Delaye, and N. Mamelle. 1999. "Mediterranean Diet, Traditional Risk Factors, and the Rate of Cardiovascular Complications After Myocardial Infarction: Final Report of the Lyon Diet Heart Study." *Circulation.* Feb. 16; 99(6):779–85.

393. Maclennan, R., F. Macrae, C. Bain, et al. 1995. "Randomized Trial of Intake of Fat, Fiber, and Beta Carotene to Prevent Colorectal Adenomas: The Australian Polyp Prevention Trial." *Journal of the National Cancer Institute.* Dec. 6; 87(23):1760–66.

394. Maegawa, H., M. Kobayashi, O. Ishibashi, Y. Takata, and Y. Shigeta. 1986. "Effect of Diet Change on Insulin Action: Difference Between Muscles and Adipocytes." *American Journal of Physiology.* Nov.; 251(5, pt. 1):E616–23.

395. Malmros, H. 1950. "The Relation of Nutrition to Health: A Statistical Study of the Effect of the War-Time on Arteriosclerosis, Cardiosclerosis, Tuberculosis, and Diabetes." *Acta Medica Scandinavica.* 246(SUPpl.):137–53'

396. Maratos-Flier, E., and J. S. Flier. 2005. "Obesity." In Kahn et al., eds., 2005, 533–45. Marble, A., P. White, R. F. Bradley, and L. P. Krall, eds. 1971. *Joslin's Diabetes Mellitus.* llth edition. Philadelphia: Lea & Febiger.

397. Marmot, M. G., S. L. Syme, A. Kagan, H. Kato, J. B. Cohen, and J. Belsky. 1975. "Epidemiologic Studies of Coronary Heart Disease and Stroke in Japanese Men living in Japan. Hawaii, and California: Prevalence of Coronary and Hypertensive Heart Disease and Associated Risk Factors." *American Journal of Epidemiology.* Dec.; 102(6): 514–25.

398. Masoro, E. J. 2003. "Subfield History: Caloric Restriction, Slowing Aging, and Extending life." *Science of Aging Knowledge Environment.* Feb. 26; 2003(8):RE2. Online at http://sageke.sciencemag.org/cgi/content/full/sageke;2003/8/re2.

399. Masoro, E. J., B. P. Yu. and H. A. Bertrand. 1982. "Action of Food Restriction in Delaying the Aging Process." *Proceedings of the National Academy of Sciences.* July; 79(13): 4239–41.

400. Mattson, F. H., and S. M. Grundy. 1985. "Comparison of Effects of Dietary Saturated, Monounsaturated, and Polyunsaturated Fatty Acids on Plasma lipids and lipoproteins in Man." *Journal of Lipid Research.* Feb.; 26(2):194–202.

401. Mauer, M. M., R. B. Harris, and T. J. Bartness. 2001. "The Regulation of Total Body Fat: Lessons Learned from lipectomy Studies." *Neuroscience & Biobehavioral Reviews.* Jan.; 25(1):15–28.

402. Mayer, J. 1976. "The Bitter Truth About Sugar." *New York Times Magazine.* June 20:26–34.

403. —. 1975a. *A Diet for Living.* New York: David McKay.

404. 1975b. "Obesity During Childhood." In Winnick. ed., 1975, 73–80.

405. —. 1974a. "By Bread Alone." *New York Times Book Review.* Dec. 15:19.

406. —. 1973a. "Diet Revolution: Basically Old Hat." *Washington Post.* April 14; F1.

407. —. 1969. "Obesity: 'Disease of Civilization.' " *Washington Post.* Nov. 30:33.

408. —. *1968. Overweight: Causes, Cost, and Control.* Englewood Cliffs, N.J.: Prentice-Hall.

409. —. 1965. "The Best Diet Is Exercise." *New York* Times *Magazine.* April 25; 34, 40, 42, 49, 50, 52, 54–5.

410. —. 1955. "Appetite and Obesity." *Atlantic.* Sept.; 58–62.

411. —. 1954. "Multiple Causative Factors in Obesity." In *Fat Metabolism,* ed. V. A. Najjar. Baltimore: Johns Hopkins University Press, 22–43.

412. —. 1953a. "Traumatic and Environmental Factors in the Etiology of Obesity." *Physiological Reviews.* Oct.; 33(4):472–508.

413. Mayer, J., N. B. Marshall. J. J. Vitale. J. H. Christensen, M. B. Mashayekhi. and F. J. Stare. 1954. "Exercise. Food Intake and Body Weight in Normal Rats and Genetically Obese Adult Mice." *American Journal of Physiology.* June; 177(3):544–48.

414. Mayer. J., and F. J. Stare. 1953. "Exercise and Weight Control." *Journal of the American Dietetic Association.* April; 29(4):340–43.

415. Mayes, P. A. 1993. "Intermediary Metabolism of Fructose." *American Journal of Clinical Nutrition.* Nov.; 58(5 supPl.):754S–65S.

416. Mayes, P. A., and K. M. Botham. 2004. "Lipid Transport & Storage." In *Harper's Illustrated Biochemistry,* 26th edition. ed. R. K. Murray. D. K. Granner, P. A. Mayes, and V. W. Rodwell (New York: Lange Medical Books/McGraw-Hill.) 205–18.

417. McClellan, W. S.. and E. F. Du Bois. 1930. "Clinical Calorimetry. XLV. Prolonged Meat Diets with a Study of Kidney Function and Ketosis." *Journal of Biological Chemistry.* July; 87(3):651–68.

418. McKeown-Eyssen, G. E., E. Bright: See, W. R. Bruce, et al. 1994. "A Randomized Trial of a Low Fat High Fibre Diet in the Recurrence of Colorectal Polyps: Toronto Polyp Prevention Group.n *Journal of Clinical Epidemiology.* May; 47(5):525–36.

419. McPherson, J. D., B. H. Shilton, and D. J. Walton. 1988. "Role of Fructose in Glycation and Cross-Linking of Proteins." *Biochemistry.* March 22; 27(6):1901–7.

420. Merkel, M., R. H. Eckel. and J. J. Goldberg. 2002. "Lipoprotein Lipase: Genetics, Lipid Uptake, and Regulation." *Journal of Lipid Research.* Dec.; 43(12):1997–2006.

421. Merrill, R. A. 1981. "Saccharin: A Regulator's View." In Crandall and Lave, eds" 1981, 153–72.

422. Michels, K. B., E. Giovannucci, K. J. Joshipura, et al. 2000. "Prospective Study of Fruit and Vegetable Consumption and Incidence of Colon and Rectal Cancers." *Journal of the National Cancer Institute.* Nov. I; 92(21):1740–52.

423. Mintz, S. W. 1986. *Sweetness and Power:* The *Place of Sugar in Modern History.* New York: Penguin Books.

424. Monnier, V. M., R. R. Kohn, and A. Cerami. 1984. "Accelerated Age-Related Browning of Human Collagen in Diabetes Mellitus." *Proceedings of the National Academy of Sciences.* Jan.; 81(2):583–87.

425. Moore, W. W. 1983. Fighting for Life: The *Story of the American Heart Association, 1911–1975.* Dallas: American Heart Association.

426. Moreira, P. I., M. A. Smith, X. Zhu, A. Nunomura, R.J. Castellani, and G. Perry. 2005. "Oxidative Stress and Neurodegeneration." *Annals of the New York Academy of Sciences.* June; 1043:545–52.

427. Mowat, F. 1978. *People of the Deer.* New York: Jove/HBJ Books.

428. Mowri, H. 0., B. Frei, and J. F. Keaney, Jr. 2000. "Glucose Enhancement of LDL Oxidation Is Strictly Metal Ion Dependent." *Free Radical Biology & Medicine.* Nov. I; 29(9):814–24.

429. Mrosovsky, N. 1985. "Cyclical Obesity in Hibernators: The Search for the Adjustable Regulator." In Hirsch and Van ltallie, eds., 1985,45–56.

430. —. 1976. "Lipid Programmes and Life Strategies in Hibernators." *American Zoologist.* 16:685–97.

431. Multiple Risk Factor Intervention Trial [MRFIT] Research Group. 1982. "Multiple Risk Factor Intervention Trial: Risk Factor Changes and Mortality Results." *JAMA.* Sept. 24; 248(12):1465–77.

432. National Center for Health Statistics [NCHS]. 2006. *Health, United States, 2006, with Chartbook on the Health of Americans.* Washington, D.C.: U.S. Government Printing Office.

433. —. 2005. *Health, United States, 2005. with Chartbook on Trends in the Health of Americans.* Washington, D.C.: U.S. Government Printing Office.

434. —. 2004. "FASTATS A to Z (2004)." Online at http://www.cdc.gov/nchs/fastats/. National Cholesterol Education Program [NCEP]. 2002. "Third Report of the National Cholesterol Education Program (NCEP) Expert Panel on Detection, Evaluation, and Treatment of High Blood Cholesterol in Adults: (Adult Treatment Panel III) Final Report." *Circulation.* Dec. 17; 106(25):3143–421.

435. National Institute of Diabetes and Digestive and Kidney Diseases [NIDDK]. 1995. The *Pima Indians: Pathfinders for Health.* NIH Publication No. 95, 3821.

436. National Research Council [NRC], Committee on Diet and Health. Food and Nutrition Board, Commission on life Sciences. 1989. *Diet and Health: Implications for Reducing Chronic Disease Risk.* Washington, D.C.: National Academy Press.

437. Neel. J. V. 1999. "The 'Thrifty Genotype' in 1998." *Nutrition Reviews.* May; 57(5, pt.2):S2–9.

438. Nestle, M. 2003. "The Ironic Politics of Obesity." *Science.* Feb. 7; 269(5608):781.

439. Nishizawa, T., I. Akaoka, Y. Nishida, Y. Kawaguchi, and E. Hayashi. 1976. "Some Factors Related to Obesity in the Japanese Sumo Wrestler." *American Journal of Clinical Nutrition*. Oct.; 29(1O):II67–'74.

440. Novartis Foundation. 2004. *Biology of IGF-1: Its Interaction with Insulin in Health and Malignant States*. Chichester, U.K.: John Wiley.

441. Novin, D., W. Wyrwicka, and G. A. Bray, eds. 1976. *Hunger. Basic Mechanisms and Clinical Implications*. New York: Raven Press.

442. Nydegger, U. R., and R. E. Butler. 1970. "Serum Lipoprotein Levels in Patients with Cancer." *Cancer Research*. Aug.; 32:1756–60.

443. Obrenovich, M. E., and V. M. Monnier. 2004. "Glycation Stimulates Amyloid Formation: *Science of Aging Knowledge Environment*. Jan. 4; No. 2:pe3. Online at http://sageke.sciencemag.org/cgi/content/full/2004/2/pe3.

444. Ogden. C. L., M. D. Carroll, L. R. Curtin, M. A. McDowell, C. J. Tabak, and K. M. Flegal. 2006. "Prevalence of Overweight and Obesity in the United States, 1999–2004." *JAMA*. April 5; 295(13):1549–55.

445. Ogden, C. L., M. D. Carroll, and K. M. Flegal. 2003. "Epidemiologic Trends in Overweight and Obesity: *Endocrinology and Metabolism Clinics of North America*. Dec.; 32(4):741–60.

446. Ohlson, M. A., W. D. Brewer, D. Kereluk, A. Wagoner, and D. C. Cederquist. 1955. "Weight Control Through Nutritionally Adequate Diets: In Eppright et aI., eds., 1955, 170–87.

447. Oliver, M. F. 1985. "Consensus or Nonsensus Conferences on Coronary Heart Disease: *Lancet*. May II; 325(8437):1087–89.

448. Orchard, T. J., M. Temprosa, R. Goldberg, et al. [Diabetes Prevention Program Research Group.) 2005. "The Effect of Metformin and Intensive Lifestyle Intervention on the Metabolic Syndrome: The Diabetes Prevention Program Randomized Trial." *Annals of Internal Medicine*. April 19; 142(8):611–19.

449. Oscai, L. B., M. M. Brown, and W. C. Miller. 1984. "Effect of Dietary Fat on Food Intake, Growth, and Body Composition in Rats." *Growth*. Winter; 48(4):415–24.

450. Osler, W. 1901. The *Principles and Practice of Medicine*. New York: D. Appleton.

451. Palgi, A., J. L. Read, I. Greenberg, M. A. Hoefer, R. R. Bistrian, and G. 1. Blackburn. 1985. "Multidisciplinary Treatment of Obesity with a Protein-Sparing Modified Fast: Results in 668 Outpatients." *American Journal of Public Health*. Oct.; 75(10):1190–94.

452. Parks, J. H., and E. Waskow. 1961. "Diabetes Among the Pima Indians of Arizona." *Arizona Medicine*. April; 18(4):99–106.

453. Pavlov, I.P. 1982. *The Digestive Glands*. Birmingham: The Classics of Medicine Library, A Division of Gryphon Editions, Ltd. [First Russian edition, 1897. English translation originally published by W.H. Thompson, 1902.]

454. Pavlov, I. P. 1955. *Selected Works*. Trans. S. Belsky. Moscow: Foreign Language Publishing House.

455. Pellet, P. L. 1987. "Problems and Pitfalls in the Assessment of Human Nutritional Status." In Harris and Ross, eds., 1987, 163–79.

456. Pennington, A. W. 1955. "Pyruvic Acid Metabolism in Obesity." *American journal of Digestive Diseases*. Feb.; 22(2):33–37.

457. —. 1954. "Treatment of Obesity: Developments of the Past 150 Years." *American Journal of Digestive Diseases*. March; 21(3):65–69.

458. —. 1953a. "Obesity: Overnutrition or Disease of Metabolism?" *American Journal of Digestive Diseases*. Sept.; 20(9):268–74.

459. —. 1953b. "Treatment of Obesity with Calorie Unrestricted Diets." *American Journal of Clinical Nutrition*. July–Aug.; 1(5):343–48.

460. —. 1953c. "A Reorientation on Obesity." *New England Journal of Medicine*. June 4; 248(23):959–64.

461. —. 1953d. "An Alternate Approach to Obesity." *American Journal of Clinical Nutrition*. Jan.; 1(2):100–106.

462. —. 1952. "Obesity." *Medical Times*. July; 80(7):389–98.

463. —. 1951a. "Caloric Requirements of the Obese." *Industrial Medicine and Surgery*. June; 20(6):267–71.

464. —. 1951b. "The Use of Fat in a Weight Reducing Diet." *Delaware State Medical Journal*. April; 23(4):79–86.

465. —. 1949. "Obesity in Industry: The Problem and Its Solution." *Industrial Medicine*. June: 259–60.

466. Peppa, M., J. Uribarri, and H. Vlassara. 2003. "Glucose, Advanced Glycation End Products, and Diabetes Complications: What Is New and What Works: Councils Voice." *Clinical Diabetes*. Oct.; 21(4):186–87.

467. Perkins, K. A. 1993. "Weight Gain Following Smoking Cessation." *Journal of Consulting and Clinical Psychology.* Oct.; 61(5):768–77.

468. Pirozzo, S., C. Summerbell, C. Cameron, and P. Glasziou. 2002. "Advice on Low-Fat Diets for Obesity." *Cochrane Database of Systematic Reviews.* No. 2:CD003640.

469. Piscatelli, R. L., G. M. Cerchio, and S. A. Kleit. 1969. "The Ketogenic Diet in the Management of Obesity." In Wilson, ed., 1969, 185–90.

470. Pollak, M. N., E. S. Schemhammer, and S. E. Hankinson. 2004. "Insulin-Like Growth Factors and Neoplasia." *Nature Reviews. Cancer.* July; 4(7):505–18.

471. Pollan, M. 2006. *Omnivore's Dilemma: A Natural History of Four Meals.* New York: Penguin Books.

472. Powles, J. 2001. "Commentary: Mediterranean Paradoxes Continue to Provoke." *International Journal of Epidemiology.* Oct.; 30(5):1076–77.

473. Powley, T. L. 1977. "The Ventromedial Hypothalamic Syndrome, Satiety, and a Cephalic Phase Hypothesis." *Psychological Review.* Jan.; 84(1):89–126.

474. Price, R. A., M. A Charles, D. J. Pettitt, and W. C. Knowler. 1993. "Obesity in Pima Indians: Large Increases Among Post-World War II Birth Cohorts." *American Journal of Physical Anthropology.* Dec.; 92(4):473–79.

475. Prior, I. A 1971. "The Price of Civilization." *Nutrition Today.* July/Aug.; 2-ll.

476. Prior, I. A, R. Beaglehole, F. Davidson, and C. E. Salmond. 1978. "The Relationships of Diabetes, Blood Lipids, and Uric Acid Levels in Polynesians." *Advances in Metabolic Disorders.* 9:241–61.

477. Prior, I. A, B. S. Rose, and F. Davidson. 1964. "Metabolic Maladies in New Zealand Maoris." *British Medical Journal.* April 25; 1(5390):1065–69.

478. Putnam, J., J. Allshouse, and L. S. Kantor. 2002. "U.S. Per Capita Food Supply Trends: More Calories, Refined Carbohydrates, and Fats." *Food Review.* Winter; 25(3):2–15.

479. Qiu, W. Q., D. M. Walsh, Z. Ye, et al. 1998. "Insulin-Degrading Enzyme Regulates Extracellular Levels of Amyloid Beta-Protein by Degradation." *Journal of Biological Chemistry.* Dec. 4; 273(49):32730–38.

480. Quintao, E., S. M. Grundy, and E. H. Ahrens. 1971. "Effects of Dietary Cholesterol on the Regulation of Total Body Cholesterol in Man." *Journal of Lipid Research.* March; 12(2):233–47.

481. Rabast, U., H. Kasper, and J. Schonborn. 1978. "Comparative Studies in Obese Subjects Fed Carbohydrate-Restricted and High Carbohydrate 1,000-Calorie Formula Diets." *Nutrition and Metabolism.* 22(5):269–77.

482. Rabast, U., J. Schonborn, and H. Kasper. 1979. "Dietetic Treatment of Obesity with Low and High-Carbohydrate Diets: Comparative Studies and Clinical Results." *International Journal of Obesity.* 1979; 3(3):201–11.

483. Rabinowitz, D., and K. L. Zierler. 1962. "Forearm Metabolism in Obesity and Its Response to Intra-Arterial Insulin: Characterization of Insulin Resistance and Evidence for Adaptive Hyperinsulinism." *Journal of Clinical Investigation.* Dec.; 41:2173–81.

484. —. 1961. "Forearm Metabolism in Obesity and Its Response to Intra-Arterial Insulin: Evidence for Adaptive Hyperinsulinism." *Lancet.* Sept. 23; 278(7204):690–92.

485. Randall, H. T. 1973. "Water, Electrolytes, and Acid-Base Balance." In Goodhart and Shils, eds., 1973, 324–61.

486. Randle, P. J., P. B. Garland, C. N. Hales, and E. A Newsholme. 1963. "The Glucose Fatty

487. Acid Cycle: Its Role in Insulin Sensitivity and the Metabolic Disturbances of Diabetes Mellitus." *Lancet.* April 13; 281(7285):787–89.

488. Ravussin, E. 2005. "Physiology: A NEAT Way to Control Weight?" *Science.* Jan. 28; 307(5709):530–31.

489. Ravussin, E., and B. A. Swinburn. 1992. "Effect of Caloric Restriction and Weight Loss on Energy Expenditure." In Wadden and Van Itallie, eds., 1992, 163–89.

490. Rea, A. M. 1983. *Once a River: Bird Life and Habitat Changes on the Middle Gila.* Tucson: University of Arizona Press.

491. Reaven, G. M. 2005. "The Insulin Resistance Syndrome: Definition and Dietary Approaches to Treatment." *Annual Review of Nutrition.* 2B91–406.

492. —. 1988. "Banting Lecture 1988: Role of Insulin Resistance in Human Disease." *Diabetes.* Dec.; 37(12):1595–607.

493. Reaven, G. M., and Y. D. Chen: 1996. "Insulin Resistance, Its Consequences, and Coronary Heart Disease: Must We Choose One Culprit?" *Circulation.* May; 93:1780–83.

494. Reaven, G. M., Y. D. Chen, J. Jeppesen, P. Maheux, and R. M. Krauss. 1993. "Insulin Resistance and HyperinsulineInia in Individuals with Small, Dense Low Density Lipoprotein Particles." *Journal of Clinical Investigation.* July; 92(1):141–46.

495. Reaven, G. M., R. L Lerner, M. P. Stem, and J. W. Farquhar. 1967. "Role of Insulin in Eridogenous HypertriglycerideInia." *Journal of Clinical Investigation.* Nov.; 46(11): 1756–67.

496. Reaven, G. M., and J. M. Olefsky. 1978. "The Role of Insulin Resistance in the Pathogenesis of Diabetes Mellitus." In *Advances in Metabolic Disorders,* vol. 9, ed. M. Miller and P. H. Bennet. New York: Academic Press, 313–33.

497. Renold, A. E., and G. F. Cahill, Jr., eds. 1965. *Handbook of Physiology. Section 5. Adipose Tissue.* Washington, D.C.: American Physiological Society.

498. Renold, A. E., O. B. Crofford, W. Stauffache1, and B. Jeanreaud. 1965. "Hormonal Control of Adipose Tissue Metabolism, with Special Reference to the Effects of Insulin." *Diabetologia.* Aug.; 1(1):4–12.

499. Reshef. L., Y. Olswang, H. Cassuto, et al. 2003. "Glyceroneogenesis and the Triglyceride/Fatty Acid Cycle." *Journal of Biological Chemistry.* Aug. 15; 278(33):30413–16.

500. Review Panel of the National Heart Institute. 1969. *Mass Field Trials of the Diet-Heart Question: Their Significance, Feasibility, and Applicability-Report of the Diet-Heart Review Panel of the National Heart Institute.* American Heart Association Monograph No. 28. American Heart Association.

501. Rittenberg, D., and R. Schoenheimer. 1937. "Deuterium as an Indicator in the Study of Intermediary Metabolism. XI. Further Studies on the Biological Uptake of Deuterium into Organic Substances, with Special Reference to Fat and Cholesterol Formation." *Journal of Biological Chemistry.* 121:235–53.

502. Rodin, J. 1987. "Weight Change Following Smoking Cessation: The Role of Food Intake and Exercise." *Addictive Behaviors. 12(4):303–17.*

503. —. 1979. "Pathogenesis of Obesity: Energy Intake and Expenditure." In Bray, ed., 1979, 37–68.

504. Rolls, B., and R. A. Barnett. 2000. The *Volumetrics Weight-Control Plan: Feel Full on Fewer Calories.* New York: HarperCollins.

505. Ross, E. B. 1987. "An Overview of Trends in Dietary Variation from Hunter-Gatherer to Modem Capitalist Societies." In Harris and Ross, eds., 1987, 7–56.

506. Rothwell, N. J., and M. J. Stock. 1981. "Thermogenesis: Comparative and Evolutionary Considerations." In Cioffi, James, and Van Itallie, eds., 1981, 335–44.

507. Rubner, M. 1982. The *Laws of Energy Conservation in Nutrition.* Ed. R. J. Joy. Trans. A. MarkoffandA. Sandri-White. New York: Academic Press. [Originally published 1902.)

508. Russell, F. 1975. *The Pima Indians.* Tucson: University of Arizona Press. [Originally published 1905.]

509. Salans, L. B., S. W. Cushman, E. S. Horton, E. Danforth, Jr., and E. A. Sims. 1974. "Hormones and the Adipocyte: Factors Influencing the Metabolic Effects of Insulin and Adrenaline." In Burland, Samuel, and Yudkin, eds., 1974, 204–16.

510. Salcedo, J., and D. Stetten, Jr. 1943. "The Turnover of Fatty Acids in the Congenitally Obese Mouse." *Journal of Biological Chemistry.* Dec.; 151(2):413–16.

511. Samaha, F. F., N. Iqubal, P. Seshadri, et al. 2003. "A Low-Carbohydrate As Compared with a Low-Fat Diet in Severe Obesity." *New England Journal of Medicine.* May 22; 348(21):2074–81.

512. Saris, W. H., S. N. Blair, M. A van Baak, et al. 2003. "How Much Physical Activity Is Enough to Prevent Unhealthy Weight Gain? Outcome of the IASO 1st Stock Conference and Consensus Statement." *Obesity Reviews.* May; 4(2):101–14.

513. Sasaki, N., R. Fukatsu, K. Tsuzuki, et al. 1998. "Advanced Glycation End Products in Alzheimer's Disease and Other Neurodegenerative Diseases." *American Journal of Pathology.* Oct.; 153(4):1149–55.

514. Schoenheimer, R. 1961. *The Dynamic State of Body Constituents.* Cambridge, Mass.: Harvard University Press.

515. Schwartz, H. 1986. *Never Satisfied: A Cultural History of Diets, Fantasies, and Fat.* New York: Doubleday.

516. Sclafani, A. 1987. "Carbohydrate, Taste, Appetite, and Obesity: An Overview." *Neuroscience & Biobehavioral Reviews.* Summer; II(2):131–53.

517. Scrimshaw, N. S., and W. Dietz. 1995. "Potential Advantages and Disadvantages of Human Obesity." In de Garine and Pollock, eds., 1995, 147–62.

518. Sears, B., and B. Lawren. 1995. *The Zone: A Dietary Road Map.* New York:HarperCollins.

519. Select Committee on Nutrition and Human Needs of the United States Senate. 1977a. *Dietary Goals for the United States.* Washington, D.C.: U.S. Government Printing Office.

520. —. 1977b. *Dietary Goals for the United States.* 2nd edition. Washington, D.C.: U.S. Government Printing Office.

521. —. 1977c. *Dietary Goals for the United States: Supplemental Views.* Washington. D.C.: U.S. Government Printing Office.

522. —. 1977d. *Cardiovascular Disease.* Vol. 2, pt. 1, of *Diet Related to* Killer *Diseases;* hearings before the Select Committee on Nutrition and Human Needs of the United States Senate, Ninety-Fifth Congress, Feb. 1 and 2, 1977. Washington, D.C.: U.S. Government Printing Office.

523. —. 1977e. *Obesity.* Vol. 2, pt. 2, of *Diet Related to* Killer *Diseases;* hearings before the Select Committee on Nutrition and Human Needs of the United States Senate, Ninety-Fifth Congress, Feb. 1 and 2,1977. Washington, D.C.: U.S. Government Printing Office.

524. —. 1977f. *Response to Dietary Goals of the United States: Re Meat.* Vol. 3 of *Diet Related to* Killer *Diseases;* hearings before the Select Committee on Nutrition and Human Needs of the United States Senate, Ninety-Fifth Congress, March 24,1977. Washington, D.C.: U.S. Government Printing Office.

525. —. 1976. *Diet Related to Killer Diseases;* hearings before the Select Committee on Nutrition and Human Needs of the United States Senate, Ninety-Fourth Congress, July 27 and 28, 1976. Washington, D.C.: U.S. Government Printing Office.

526. —. 1973a. *Sugar in Diet, Diabetes, and Heart Disease.* Hearing Before the Select Committee on Nutrition and Human Needs of the United States Senate, Ninety-Third Congress, pt. 2, April 30, May 1 and 2, 1973. Washington, D.C.: U.S. Government Printing Office.

527. —. 1973b. *Obesity and Fad Diets;* hearing Before the Select Committee on Nutrition and Human Needs of the United States Senate, Ninety-Third Congress, pt. I, April 12, 1973. Washington, D.C.: U.S. Government Printing Office.

528. Shafrir, E. 1991. "Metabolism of Disaccharides and Monosaccharides with Emphasis on Sucrose and Fructose and Their Lipogenic Potential." In Gracey, Kretchmer, and Rossi, eds., 1991, 131–52.

529. —. 1985. "Effect of Sucrose and Fructose on Carbohydrate and Lipid Metabolism and the Resulting Consequences." In *Regulation of Carbohydrate Metabolism,* vol. 2, ed. R. Beitner. Boca Raton, Fla.: CRC Press, 95–14°.

530. Shen, M. M., R. M. Krauss, F. T. Lindgren, and T. M. Forte. 1981. "Heterogeneity of Serum Low Density Lipoproteins in Normal Human Subjects." *Journal of Lipid Research.* Feb.; 22(2):236–44.

531. Shen, S. W., G. M. Reaven, and J. W. Farquhar. 1970. "Comparison of Impedance to Insulin-Mediated Glucose Uptake in Normal Subjects and in Subjects with Latent Diabetes." *Journal of Clinical Investigation.* Dec.; 49(12):2151–60.

532. Simpson, R G., A. Benedetti, G. M. Grodsky, J. H. Karam, and P. H. Forsham. 1968. "Early Phase of Insulin Release." *Diabetes.* Nov.; 17(11):684–92.

533. Sims, E. A. 1976. "Experimental Obesity, Dietary-Induced Thermogenesis, and Their Clinical Implications." *Clinics in Endocrinology* 6[*Metabolism.* July; 5(2):377–95.

534. Sims, E. A., G. A. Bray, E. Danforth, Jr., et al. 1974. "Experimental Obesity in Man. VI. The Effect of Variations in Intake of Carbohydrate on Carbohydrate, lipid, and Cortisol Metabolism." *Hormone and Metabolic Research Supplement.* 4:70–77.

535. Sims, E. A., and E. Danforth, Jr. 1987. "Expenditure and Storage of Energy in Man." *Journal of Clinical Investigation.* April; 79(4):1019–25.

536. —. 1974. "Role of Insulin in Obesity." *Israeli Journal of Medical Sciences.* Oct.; 10(10):1222–29.

537. Sims, E. A., E. Danforth, Jr., E. S. Horton, G. A. Bray, J. A. Glennon, and L B. Salans. 1973. "Endocrine and Metabolic Effects of Experimental Obesity in Man." *Recent Progress in Hormone Research.* 29:457–96.

538. Sims, E. A., and E. S. Horton. 1968. "Endocrine and Metabolic Adaptation to Obesity and Starvation." *American Journal of Clinical Nutrition.* Dec.; 21(12):1455–70.

539. Sinclair, U. 2003. *The Jungle.* Tucson: Sharp Press. [Originally published 1906]

540. Singh, R, A. Barden, T. Mori, and L. Beilin. 2001. "Advanced Glycation End-Products: A Review." *Diabetologia.* Feb.; 44(2):129–46.

541. Smith, C. J., E. M. Manahan, and S. G. Pablo. 1994. "Food Habit and Cultural Changes Among the Pima Indians." In Joe and Young, eds., 1994, 407–33.

542. Smith, M. A., P. L Richey, S. Taneda, et al. 1994. "Advanced Maillard Reaction End Products, Free Radicals, and Protein Oxidation in Alzheimer's Disease." *Annals of the* New *York Academy of Sciences.* June 7; 91(12):5710–14.

543. Sondike, S. B., N. Copperman, and M. S. Jacobson. 2003. "Effects of a Low-Carbohydrate Diet on Weight Loss and Cardiovascular Risk Factor in Overweight Adolescents." *Journal of Pediatrics.* March; 142(3):253–58.

544. Spicer, E. H. 1962. *Cycles of Conquest:* The *Impact of Spain, Mexico, and the United States on the Indians of the Southwest,* 1533–1960. Tucson: University of Arizona Press.

545. Stamler. J. 1967. *Lectures on Preventive Cardiology.* New York: Grune & Stratton.

546. —. 1962. "The Early Detection of Heart Disease: In *Heart Disease Control,* ed. F. W. Reynolds. Ann Arbor: University of Michigan School of Public Health Continued Edu cation Series no. 97,48–71.

547. Stamler. J.. D. M. Berkson. and H. A. Lindberg. 1972. "Risk Factors: Their Role in the Etiology and Pathogenesis of the Atherosclerotic Diseases: In The *Pathogenesis of Atherosclerosis,* eds. R. W. Wissler and J. C. Geer. Baltimore: Williams & Wilkins, 41–119.

548. Stamler. J., D. Wentworth, and J. D. Neaton. 1986. "Is Relationship Between Serum Cholesterol and Risk of Premature Death from Coronary Heart Disease Continuous and Graded? Findings in 356,222 Primary Screenees of the Multiple Risk Factor Intervention Trial (MRFIT)." *JAMA.* Nov. 28; 256(20):2823–28.

549. Stare, F. J. 1987. *Harvard's Department of Nutrition,* 1942–1986. Norwell. Mass.: Christopher Publishing House.

550. Stefansson. V. 1946. *Not by Bread Alone.* New York: Macmillan, 1936. "Adventures in Diet. Reprint from *Harper's Monthly Magazine.* Chicago: Institute of American Meat Packers.

551. Stein, J. H., K. M. West. J. M. Robey. D. F. Tirador, and G. W. McDonald. 1965. "The High Prevalence of Abnormal Glucose Tolerance in the Cherokee Indians of North Carolina.. *Archives of Internal Medicine.* Dec.; 116(6):842–45.

552. Steinberg, D. 2005. "An Interpretive History of the Cholesterol Controversy. Part II. The Early Evidence linking Hypercholesterolemia to Coronary Disease in Humans." *Journal of Lipid Research.* Feb.; 46(2):179–90.

553. —. 1997. "Low Density lipoprotein Oxidation and Its Pathobiological Significance." *Journal of Biological Chemistry.* Aug. 22; 272(34):20963–66.

554. Steinberg, D., and M. Vaughan. 1965. "Release of Free Fatty Acids from Adipose Tissue in-Vitro in Relation to Rates of Triglyceride Synthesis and Degradation." In Renold and Cahill, eds., 1965, 335–47.

555. Stene, J. A., and I. L. Roberts. 1928. "A Nutrition Study on an Indian Reservation." *Journal of the American Dietetic Association.* March; 3(4):215–22.

556. Steward, H. L., M. C. Bethea, S. S. Andrews, and L. A. Balart. 1998. *Sugar Busters! Cut Sugar to Trim Fat.* New York: Ballantine Books.

557. Stitt, A. W. 2001. Advanced Glycation: An Important Pathological Event in Diabetic and Age Related Ocular Disease." *British Journal of Ophthalmology.* June; 85(6):746–53.

558. Stitt, A. W., R. Bucala, and H. Vlassara. 1997. "Atherogenesis and Advanced Glycation: Promotion, Progression, and Prevention. *Annals of the New York Academy of Sciences.* April 15; 8n:n5–27, 127–29.

559. Stock, A. L., and J. Yudkin. 1970. "Nutrient Intake of Subjects on Low Carbohydrate Diet Used in Treatment of Obesity." *American Journal of Clinical Nutrition.* July; 23(7): 948–52.

560. Stock, M., and N. Rothwell. 1982. *Obesity and Leanness: Basic Aspects.* New York: John Wiley. Stockton, W. 1989. "When Exercise Isn't Enough." *New York Times.* Feb. 20; C11. Stolberg, S. G. 1999. "Fiber Does Not Help Prevent Colon Cancer, Study Finds." *New York* Times. Jan. 21; A14.

561. Stout, R. W. 1970. "Development of Vascular Lesions in Insulin-Treated Animals Fed a Normal Diet." *British Medical Journal.* Sept. 19; 3(5724):685–87.

562. Stout, R. W., E. L. Bierman, and R. Ross. 1975. "Effect of Insulin on the Proliferation of Cultured Primate Arterial Smooth Muscle Cells." *Circulation Research.* Feb.; 36(2): 319–27.

563. Stout, R. W., and J. Vallance-Owen. 1969. "Insulin and Atheroma." *Lancet.* May 31; 293(76°5):1078–80.

564. Strittmatter, W. J., A. M. Saunders, D. Schmechel, et al. 1993. "Apolipoprotein E: High-Avidity Binding to Beta-Amyloid and Increased Frequency of Type 4 Allele in Late-Onset Familial Alzheimer Disease.' *Proceedings of the National Academy of Sciences.* March I; 90(5):1977–81.

565. Stunkard, A. J., ed. 1980. *Obesity.* Philadelphia: W. B. Saunders.

566. —. 1980. "Introduction and Overview.' In Stunkard, ed., 1980, 1–24.

567. —. 1976a. "Obesity and Social Environment.' In Howard, ed., 1976, 178–90

568. —. 1976b. *The Pain of Obesity.* Palo Alto, Calif: Bull Publishing.

569. —. 1976c. "Studies on TOPS: A Self-Help Group for Obesity." In Bray, ed., 1976b, 387–92.

570. —. 1973. "The Obese: Background and Programs." In Mayer, ed., 1973, 29–36.

571. Stunkard, A., and M. McClaren-Hume. 1959. "The Results of Treatment for Obesity: A Review of the Literature and a Report of a Series.' *Archives of Internal Medicine.* Jan.; 103(1):79–85.

572. Stunkard, A. J., and T. A. Wadden, eds. 1993. *Obesity: Theory and Therapy.* 2nd edition. New York: Raven Press.

573. Suarez, G., J. D. Etlinger, J. Maturana, and D. Weitman. 1995. "Fructated Protein Is More Resistant to ATP-Dependent Proteolysis Than Glucated Protein Possibly as a Result of Higher Content of Maillard Fluorophores." *Archives of Biochemistry and Biophysics.* Aug. I; 321(1):209–13.

574. Suarez, G., R. Rajaram, O. 1. Oronsky, and M. A. Gawinowicz. 1989. "Nonenzymatic Glycation of Bovine Serum Albumin by Fructose (Fructation): Comparison with the Maillard Reaction Initiated by Glucose. *Journal of Biological Chemistry.* March 5; 264(7):3674–79.

575. Sugarman, C. 1999. "Eat Fat, Get Thin? Dieters on Protein-Rich Regimens Report Great Success, but Some Doctors Question the Safety of These Low-Carb Plans. *Washington Post.* Nov. 23; Z10.

576. —. 1989. "Experts Agree: Eat More Fruit, Vegetables." *Washington Post.* March 2; AI. Sullivan, P. 2004. "Ancel Keys, K Ration Creator, Dies." *Washington Post.* Nov. 24; AI.

577. Surkan, P. J., C. C. Hsieh, A. 1. Johansson, P. W. Dickman, and S. Cnattingius. 2004. "Reasons for Increasing Trends in Large for Gestational Age Births." *Obstetrics & Gynecology.* Oct.; 104(4):720–26.

578. Susic, D., J. Varagic, J. Ahn, and E. D. Frohlich. 2004. "Crosslink Breakers: A New Approach to Cardiovascular Therapy. " *Current Opinion in Cardiology.* July; 19(4):336–40.

579. Swanson, J. E., D. C. Laine, W. Thomas, and J. P. Bantle. 1992. "Metabolic Effects of Dietary Fructose in Healthy Subjects." *American Journal of Clinical Nutrition.* April; 55(4):851–56.

580. Sytkowski, P. A., W. B. Kannel, and R. B. D'Agostino. 1990. "Changes in Risk Factors and the Decline in Mortality from Cardiovascular Disease: The Framingham Heart Study." *New England Journal of Medicine.* June 7; 322(23):1635–41.

581. Szanto, S., and J. Yudkin. 1969. "The Effect of Dietary Sucrose on Blood Lipids, Serum Insulin, Platelet Adhesiveness, and Body Weight in Human Volunteers." *Postgraduate Medical Journal.* Sept.; 45(527):602–7.

582. Tanzi, R. E., and A. B. Parson. 2000. *Decoding Darkness: The Search for the Genetic Causes of Alzheimer's Disease.* Cambridge, Mass.: Perseus Publishing.

583. Tappy, L., and E. Jequier. 1993. "Fructose and Dietary Thermogenesis." *American Journal of Clinical Nutrition.* Nov.; 58(5 suppl.):766s–70s.

584. Tarnower, H., and S. S. Baker. 1978. *The Complete Scarsdale Medical Diet.* New York: Bantam Books.

585. Task Force Sponsored by the American Society for Clinical Nutrition. 1979. "The Evidence Relating Six Dietary Factors to the Nations Health." *American Journal of Clinical Nutrition.* 32(suppl.):2621–748.

586. Taubs, G. 2007. *Good Calories, Bad Calories.* New York: Alfred A. Knopf.

587. —. 1996. "Looking for the Evidence in Medicine." *Science.* April 5; 272(5258):22–24.

588. Teng, B., G. R. Thompson, A. D. Sniderman, T. M. Forte, R. M. Krauss, and P. O. Kwiterovich, Jr. 1983. "Composition and Distribution of Low Density Lipoprotein Fractions in HyperApoBetalipoproteinemia, Normolipidemia, and Familial Hypercholesterolemia." *Proceedings of the National Academy of Sciences.* Nov.; 80(21): 6662–66.

589. Thomas, B. M., and A. T. Miller. 1958. "Adaptation to Forced Exercise in the Rat." *American Journal of Physiology.* May; 193(2):350–54.

590. Thompson, L., and S. Squires. 1987. "What You Should Know, How You Should Eat, When You Should Worry: Cholesterol Survival Guide." *Washington Post.* Oct. 20; Z14. Thorpe. G. L. 1957. "Treating Overweight Patients." *JAMA.* Nov. 16; 165(11):1361–65. Tolchin, M. 1959. "Helping the Overweight Child." *New York* Times *Magazine.* Oct. II; 62–64.

591. Toufexis. A. 1988. "The Food You Eat May Kill You." Time. Aug. 8. Online at http://www.time.com/time/magazine/article/ 0.9171,968077 ,00.htrnl.

592. Trowell, H. C., and D. P. Burkitt, eds. 1981. *Western Diseases: Their Emergence and Prevention.* London: Edward Arnold.

593. U.K Department of Health. 1998. *Nutritional Aspects of the Development of Cancer. Report of the Working Group on Diet and Cancer of the Committee on Medical Aspects of Food and Nutritional* Policy. *Report on Health and Social Subjects* 48. London: The Stationery Office.

594. —. 1994. *Nutritional Aspects of Cardiovascular Disease. Report of the Cardiovascular Review Group of the Committee on Medical Aspects of Food* Policy. *Report on Health and Social Subjects* 46. London: Her Majesty's Stationery Office.

595. —. 1989. *Dietary Sugars and Human Disease. Report of the Panel on Dietary Sugars. Committee on Medical Aspects of Food* Policy. *Report on Health and Social Subjects 37.* London: Her Majesty's Stationery Office.

596. U.S. Department of Agriculture (USDA). n.d. Nutrient Database for Standard Reference. Online at http://www.nal.usda.gov/fnic/cgi-bin/ nu_search.pl.

597. —. 2000. "Major Trends in U.S. Food Supply, 1909–99'" *FoodReview.* Jan.–April; 23(1):8–15.

598. —. 1992. "The Food Guide Pyramid." *Home and Garden Bulletin* No. 252. Washington, D.C.: U.S. Government Printing Office.

599. —. *1953. Consumption of Food in the United States,* 1909–1952. Agriculture Handbook No. 62. Washington, D.C.: USDA Bureau of Agricultural Economics.

600. U.S. Department of Agriculture and U.S. Department of Health, Education, and Welfare [HEW]. 1980. "Nutrition and Your Health: Dietary Guidelines for Americans." *Home and Garden Bulletin.* No. 228. Washington, D.C.: U.S. Department of Agriculture.

601. U.S. Department of Health and Human Services [USDHHS]. 2001. *The Surgeon General's* Call *to Action to Prevent and Decrease Overweight and Obesity,* 2001. Washington D.C.: U.S. Government Printing Office.

602. —. 1988. *The Surgeon General's Report on Nutrition and Health.* Washington, D.C. U.S. Government Printing Office.

603. U.S. Department of Health and Human Services and U.S. Department of Agriculture. *2005. Dietary Guidelines for Americans,* 2005. 6th edition. Washington, D.C.: U.S. Government Printing Office.

604. Van Itallie, T. B. 1980a. "Dietary Approaches to the Treatment of Obesity." In Stunkard, ed., 1980, 249–61.

605. —. 1980b. "Diets for Weight Reduction: Mechanisms of Action and Physiologic Effects." In Bray, ed., 1980, 15–24.

606. —. 1979. "Conservative Approaches to Treatment." In Bray, ed., 1979, 164–78.

607. —. 1978. "Dietary Approaches to the Treatment of Obesity." *Psychiatric Clinics of North America.* Dec.; 1(3):609–20. [Also referenced as A. J. Stunkard, ed., *Obesity: Basic Mechanisms and Treatment* (Philadelphia: W. B. Saunders, 1978))

608. Van Itallie, T. B., and T. H. Nufert. 2003. "Ketones: Metabolism's Ugly Duckling." *Nutrition Review.* Oct.; 61(10):327–41.

609. Vaselli, J. R., M. P. Cleary, and T. B. Van Itallie. 1984. "Obesity." In Olson et al., eds., 1984, 35–56.

610. Vitek, M. P., K. Bhattacharya, J. M. Glendening, et al. 1994. "Advanced Glycation End Products Contribute to Amyloidosis in Alzheimer Disease." *Proceedings of the National Academy of Sciences.* May 24; 91(11):4766–70.

611. Wadden, T. A., A. J. Stunkard, K. D. Brownell, and S. C. Day. 1985. "A Comparison of Two Very-low-Calorie Diets: Protein-Sparing-Modified Fast Versus Protein-Formula Liquid Diet." *American Journal of Clinical Nutrition.* March; 41(3):533–39.

612. Wadden, T. A., and T. B. Van Itallie, eds. 1992. *Treatment of the Seriously Obese Patient.* New York: Guilford Press.

613. Walker, A. R., P. E. Cleaton-Jones, and B. D. Richardson. 1978. "Is Sugar Good for You?" *South African Medical Journal.* Oct. 7; 54(15):589–90.

614. Waterlow, J. C. 1986. "Metabolic Adaptation to Low Intakes of Energy and Protein." *Annual Review of Nutrition.* 6:495–526.

615. Webb, G. 1992. *A Pima Remembers.* Tucson: University of Arizona Press. [Originally published 1959]

616. Weinert, B. T., and P. S. Timiras. 2003. "Theories of Aging." *Journal of Applied Physiology.* Oct.; 95(4):1706–16.

617. Wessen, A. 2001. "Ian Prior and the Tokelau Island Migrant Studies: In *The Health of Pacific Societies: Ian Prior's Life and Work* (Aoteroa, N.Z.: Steele Roberts), 16–25.

618. West, K. M. 1981. "North American Indians: In Trowell and Burkitt, eds., 1981, 129–37.

619. Whelan, E. M., and F. J. Stare. 1983. *The One-Hundred-Percent Natural, Purely Organic, Cholesterol-Free, Megavitamin, Low-Carbohydrate Nutrition Hoax.* New York: Atheneum.

620. Will, J. C., and T. Byers. 1996. "Does Diabetes Mellitus Increase the Requirement for Vitamin C?" *Nutrition Reviews.* July; 54(7):193–202.

621. Willett, W. C. 2001. *Eat, Drink, and Be Healthy: The Harvard Medical School Guide to Healthy Eating.* New York: Simon & Schuster.

622. Willett, W. C., F. Sacks, A. Trichopoulos, et al. 1995. "Mediterranean Diet Pyramid: A Cultural Model for Healthy Eating." *American Journal of Clinical Nutrition.* June; 61(6suppl.):1402S–6S.

623. Witztum, J. 1., and D. Steinberg. 1981. "Role of Oxidized Low Density Lipoprotein in Atherogenesis." *Journal of Clinical Investigation.* Dec.; 88(6):1785–92.

624. Wolever, T. M. 1997. "The Glycemic Index: Flogging a Dead Horse?" *Diabetes Care.* March; 20(3):452–56.

625. World Health Organization. 2006. "The World Health Organization Notes the Women's Health Initiative Diet Modification Trial, but Reaffirms That the Fat Content of Your Diet Does Matter." Downloaded Feb. 16, 2006. Online at http://www.who.int/nmh/media/Response_Statement_16_feb_06F.pd£

626. —. 2004. "Global Strategy on Diet, Physical Activity and Health, Obesity and Overweight." Downloaded March 25, 2005. Online at http://www.who.int/dietphysical activity /publications/facts/obesity/ en/.

627. —. 2003. "Nutrition in Transition: Globalization and Its Impact on Nutritional Patterns and Diet-Related Diseases. Updated Wed. Sept. 3, 2003. Online at http://www . who.int/nut/trans.htm.

628. Wu, Y., S. Yakar, L. Zhao, 1. Hennighausen, and D. LeRoith. 2002. "Circulating InsulinLike Growth Factor-I Levels Regulate Colon Cancer Growth and Metastasis: *Cancer Research.* Feb. 15; 62(4):1030–35.

629. Yalow, R. S., and S. A. Berson. 1960. "Immunoassay of Endogenous Plasma Insulin in Man: *Journal of Clinical Investigation.* July; 39:1157–75.

630. Yalow, R. S., S. M. Glick, J. Roth, and S. A. Berson. 1965. "Plasma Insulin and Growth Hormone Levels in Obesity and Diabetes." *Annals of the New York Academy of Sciences.* Oct. 8; 131(1):357–73.

631. Yan, S. D., X. Chen, A. M. Schmidt, et al. 1994. "Glycated Tau Protein in Alzheimer Disease: A Mechanism for Induction of Oxidant Stress: *Proceedings of the National Academy of Sciences.* Aug. 2; 91(16):7787–91.

632. Yancy, W. S., Jr., M. K. Olsen, J. R. Guyton, R. P. Bakst, and E. C. Westman. 2004. "A LowCarbohydrate, Ketogenic Diet Versus a Low-Fat Diet to Treat Obesity and Hyperlipidemia: A Randomized, Controlled Trial." *Annals of Internal Medicine.* May 18; 140(10):769–77.

633. Young. C. M., I. Ringler, and B. J. Greer. 1953. "Reducing and Post-Reducing Maintenance on the Moderate Fat Diet: Metabolic Studies: *Journal of the American Dietetic Association.* Sept.; 29(9):890–96.

634. Young, R. A. 1976. "Fat, Energy and Mammalian Survival." *American Zoologist.* 16:699–710.

635. Yudkin, J. 1986. *Pure, White, and Deadly.* Revised edition. New York: Viking.

636. —. 1974. "The Low-Carbohydrate Diet: In Burland, Samuel. and Yudkin, eds.. 1974, 271–80.

637. —. 1972a. *Pure, White, and Deadly.* London: Davis-Poynter.

638. —. 1972b. *Sweet and Dangerous.* New York: P. H. Wyden.

639. —. 1972C. "The low-Carbohydrate Diet in the Treatment of Obesity: *Postgraduate Medical journal.* May; 51(5):151–54.

640. —. 1959. "The Causes and Cure of Obesity: *Lancet.* Dec. 19; 274(7u2):U35–38.

641. —. 1958. This *Slimming Business.* London: MacGibbon and Kee.

642. —. 1957. "Diet and Coronary Thrombosis: Hypothesis and Fact: *Lancet.* July 27; 270(6987):155–62.

643. Yudkin, J., and M. Carey. 1960. "The Treatment of Obesity by the 'High-Fat' Diet: The Inevitability of Calories.. *Lancet.* Oct. 29; 276(7157):939–41.

644. Yudkin, J., V. V. Kakkar, and S. Szanto. 1969. "Sugar Intake, Serum Insulin and Platelet Adhesiveness in Men with and Without Peripheral Vascular Disease.. *Postgraduate Medical Journal.* Sept.; 45(527):608–11.

645. Zierler, K. L., and D. Rabinowitz. 1964. "Effect of Very Small Concentrations of Insulin on Forearm Metabolism: Persistence of Its Action on Potassium and Free Fatty Acids Without Its Effect on Glucose.. *Journal of Clinical Investigation.* May; 43:950–62.

646. Zukel, W. J., O. Paul, and H. W. Schnaper. 1981. "The Multiple Risk Factor Intervention Trial (MRFIT). I. Historical Perspective.. *Preventive Medicine.* July; 10(4):387:–401.

INDEX

MORE INFORMATION

WWW.FACTOR4HEALTH.COM
More information about power amino acids® and the Factor4 weight loss study

WWW.IMPROVEWORLDHEALTH.ORG
More information about the mission of a non-profit organization to improve world health with power amino acids®

WWW.DRGEORGESCHEELE.COM
More information about the author including the author's past achievements

BLOGGING SITES

WWW.WEIGHTCONTROL4LIFE.COM

FACTOR4 WELLNESS PROGRAM

The Factor4 Wellness Program sends out weekly information on essential health care to its members. The program includes four weekly themes that rotate on a monthly basis: These themes are *Healthy Lifestyles; Weight Control; Metabolic Health; and Anti-Aging.*

To become a free member of the Factor4 Wellness Program, register at www.factor4health.com

MEET DR. SCHEELE,
CREATOR OF FACTOR4 WEIGHT
CONTROL®

Dr. George A. Scheele, world lecturer, physician and founder of NovaLife, Inc., in La Jolla, California, has recently introduced **Factor4 Weight Control**®, a delicious nutritional shake, for treatment of the four nutritional traps in overweight conditions and obesity: **the Taste Trap, the Vanity Trap, the Food Swing Trap, and the Sedentary Trap**

Factor4 Weight Control® provides all the nutrients that your body needs, including vitamins, minerals, micronutrients, health-plus proteins™ and power amino acids®, to (i) restore nutritional health, (ii) control appetite and (iii) burn fat.

Power Amino Acids® and **Health-Plus Proteins**™ contained in Factor4 Weight Control® are critically important in today's sedentary society to provide the essential nutrients (essential amino acids) that are needed for nutritional health, mental health and weight control. These power supplements will enhance your feelings of "wellness" in up to 50 different ways in the eight (8) major health systems of the body.

Schooled in the Ivy League and trained in Medicine at Johns Hopkins and the University of California at San Francisco, Dr. Scheele served as Professors of Medicine at The Rockefeller University, Yale University School of Medicine and Harvard Medical School. A pioneer in the development of the fields of Cell and Molecular Biology and their impact on understanding chronic human diseases, he participated in work that won two Nobel Prizes in Medicine awarded in 1974 and 1999.

In a series of celebrated papers published between 1975 and 1995, Dr. Scheele and his collaborators invented new techniques that ultimately "cracked the code" in understanding the "molecular secrets" for how Power Amino Acids® and Health-Plus Proteins™ treat amino acid and protein deficiency disorders associated with overweight conditions and obesity.

As a leader in nutritional science and a pioneer in medical research, Dr. Scheele's passion has always been to "**Make the World a Better Place**". After moving to La Jolla in 1998, he founded NovaLife, Inc. and utilized his vast experience to develop superior health-care products for individuals living in today's fast-paced world. His recent book, entitled *THE OBESITY CURE: Weight Control, Metabolic Health and Revitalized Youth with Power Amino Acids*, explains the link between protein health and normal body weight.

ADDITIONAL PRAISE FOR *THE OBESITY CURE*

Before I read Dr. Scheele's book, The Obesity Cure, *I could not understand why I would eat three meals a day and still snack to satisfy my appetite in between meals. I could not understand why I was 50 pounds overweight and could not take off another pound. Through* The Obesity Cure, *I learned that we all suffer from addictive taste disorders, largely due to the excessive quantities of refined sugars that the food industry adds to most processed foods. Through the compelling logic of Dr. Scheele's book I learned how to "tame" my appetite and rebalance my metabolism to achieve normal body weight after all these years.*

Armour Black
Palm Springs, California

In The Obesity Cure *Dr. Scheele explains, for the first time, why popular diets do not work and takes a global approach to understanding obesity and metabolic disease. The way this book explains the vulnerability of the food chain and its effects on body weight and metabolic health represents a real breakthrough in health care. Thanks to this extraordinary book I have found innumerable ways to make delicious shakes and smoothies that reduce my appetite and increase my energy for long periods of time. This is* <u>THE OBESITY CURE</u>.

Carol Wagner
Baltimore, MD

I can heartedly recommend The Obesity Cure. *Dr. Scheele's new book on nutrition, metabolic health and weight control makes good common sense. No other author has brought all the facts and observations collected over the last century together in a way that is easy to understand and a joy to read. This book is artfully written and compelling in its logic. Seldom does one see so many lose ends pulled together, deconstructed and redirected into a compelling approach to treat an epidemic that is destroying the health of our country. Bravo to the author for providing* The Obesity Cure.

Mary Krebill
Poway, California

Dr. Scheele's strategy, expressed in The Obesity Cure, *to use natural amino acids to harness the body's natural feedback mechanisms to boost energy, build muscle and shed fat suggests that Dr. Scheele's long career in studying dietary disease in animals and humans has given him a unique ability to solve America's #1 metabolic disease: obesity. The Obesity Cure is full of discoveries that can help men and women avoid the metabolic traps that lead to overweight disorders, metabolic disease and accelerated aging.*

Georgeann Crawford
South Carolina

More than any other health book in today's market, The Obesity Cure *explains, with clear compelling logic, why America is suffering from the "Battle of the Bulge" and what must be done to stop the epidemics of both obesity and metabolic disease. The solution revealed in* The Obesity Cure *is the use of Power Amino Acids to reduce appetite, build muscle, burn fat and boost energy. The genius of the book is the way that Dr. Scheele explains the vulnerability of the food chain that leads to diet-related deficiencies in positive-charged amino acids, proteins and metabolic pathways, which cause unwanted weight gains. Dr. Scheele further explains how Power Amino Acids, comprised of essential, positive-charged and satiety amino acids, have the power to tame appetite and normalize body weight. This book is a triumph of reason and discovery over disease and should be read by every American who suffers from metabolic disease and obesity.*

Chris Walker
New York City

The Obesity Cure *has changed my life in the most dramatic fashion. In 6 months my body weight fell from 267 pounds to 201 pounds. That is 66 pounds lost for good. My waist was reduced from a size 44 to a comfortable size 34. I have never seen a strategy that loses weight this efficiently and a system that can thin-down or bulk-up at will! Dr. Scheele's book explains why vulnerabilities in the food chain can lead to metabolic disease, including obesity; high cholesterol, sugar and blood pressure; type 2 diabetes; cardiovascular disease; certain cancers; gallbladder disease; liver disease; and kidney disease. This book is so illuminating in a field of darkness that it provides a beacon of light for all Americans who suffer from chronic disease. This book is a "must-read." It will change your life forever.*

Dale Lawson
Carlsbad, California

I came to know Dr. Scheele because I have suffered for years from high cholesterol and excess weight. Initially my cholesterol could only be lowered with Lipitor. However, I was unfortunate to suffer from the harmful side-effects of Lipitor, including the myalgia syndrome, sharp muscular pains 24/7. I had nowhere to turn. My doctor advised me to try protein powders and I tried every powder I could find. However, the only powder that worked for me was Factor4 Weight Control®, a high-nutrient, low-calorie nutritional shake, containing Power Amino Acids that Dr. Scheele formulated several years ago. Although I still have some muscle pain, it has been reduced by 70% and my need for Lipitor has dropped significantly. I am so grateful for Dr. Scheele's new discovery that Factor4 is my constant companion. Now Dr. Scheele has explained his new technologies in The Obesity Cure, *which is the most outstanding book on the market today. Not only does Dr. Scheele explain why we gain unwanted weight, but how to improve nutrition to lose unwanted weight without counting calories, points or suffering from constant hunger. Kudos to Dr. Scheele and* The Obesity Cure.

Laura Bricker
Coronado, California

I was pleasantly surprised at the clarity and logic that is so artfully presented in The Obesity Cure. *For the first time I could understand how toxic refined sugars, whether high fructose corn syrup or sucrose (table sugar), are to the body. I could finally understand how sugar toxicity leads to obesity and cardiovascular disease. I could understand why fructose is more toxic than glucose. But the most important part of the book explains how Power Amino Acids tame appetite, metabolic disease and overweight diseases. For the first time I learned about the realities of the food chain and the importance of fermented foods in other cultures. For the first time I now have complete control over the health of my body, which includes body energy and weight. So simple…so elegant…so timely…*The Obesity Cure.

Leticia Morgan
Chula Vista, California

Dr. Scheele's latest book, entitled The Obesity Cure, *explains for the first time, in simple language, how to achieve normal body weight and super-charged health, particularly as we begin to age. The concepts presented in this book on the toxicity of refined sugars and the beneficial effects of essential, positive-charged and satiety amino acids (what Dr. Scheele refers to as Power Amino Acids) in curbing appetite for carbs and restoring metabolic health and normal body weight, is masterful. This is* The BOOK *to follow in revitalizing health in today's America. Do not waste a minute…purchase this game-changing book NOW. Following the concepts introduced in* The Obesity Cure, *I lost 120 pounds in 9 months as I reduced my weight from 334 to 214 pounds. When I lose another 34 pounds, I will have reestablished the Marine Corps body that I possessed 30 years ago. Need I say more!*

James Hill
Alabama